AF879650

The Peptides Blue Book

Discover the Latest Research Behind Optimal Health, Muscle Growth, and Anti-Aging Strategies (150 Peptides + Dosage Guide)

Copyright by Newstone Publishing - All rights reserved.

Printed in the United States of America.

Newstone Publishing does not endorse any political or religious statement via this publication.

This book is geared towards providing precise and reliable information about the topic.

This publication is sold with the idea that the publisher is not required to render any accounting, officially or otherwise, or any other qualified services. If further advice is necessary, contacting a legal and/or financial professional is recommended.

From a Declaration of Principles that was accepted and approved equally by a Committee of the American Bar Association and a Committee of Publishers' Associations.

In no way is it legal to reproduce, duplicate, or transmit any part of this document, either by electronic means, or in printed format. Recording this publication is strictly prohibited, and any storage of this document is not allowed unless with written permission from the publisher. All rights reserved.

The information provided herein is stated to be truthful and consistent, in that any liability, in terms of inattention or otherwise, by any usage or abuse of any policies, processes, or directions contained within, is the solitary and utter responsibility of the recipient reader. Under no circumstances will any legal responsibility or blame be held against the publisher for any reparation, damages, or monetary loss due to the information herein, either directly or indirectly.

Respective authors own all copyrights not held by the publisher.

The information herein is offered for informational purposes solely, and is universally presented as such. The information herein is also presented without contract or any type of guarantee or assurance.

The trademarks presented are done so without any consent, and this publication of the trademarks is without permission or backing by the trademark owners. All trademarks and brands within this book are thus for clarifying purposes only and are owned by the owners themselves, and are not affiliated otherwise with this document.

Table of Contents

****The audiobook and digital flash cards can be accessed via a QR code that is located on the last page of this book. If the QR code does not work for you, please contact mbenterprise2016@gmail.com and mention the title of this book.**

Background

Peptides are one of the most powerful tools in modern health and performance optimization. These short chains of amino acids act as signaling molecules in the body. They influence everything from metabolism and muscle growth to cognitive function and immune resilience. Although peptides have been used in medicine for decades, mainly in hormone therapy and regenerative medicine, recent advancements have expanded their applications to longevity, fat loss, brain health, and even aesthetics.

This guide serves as an essential resource for anyone who wants to understand and harness the potential of peptides safely and effectively. Whether you're an athlete who works toward peak performance, a biohacker in search of cutting-edge anti-aging strategies, or a medical professional who wants to enhance patient outcomes, this book provides an in-depth look into the world of peptides.

In this introduction, we will explore the fundamental types of peptides, including:

- **Metabolic Peptides** – Burn more fat and regulate appetite.
- **Growth and Repair Peptides** – Promote muscle recovery and tissue regeneration.
- **Nootropic Peptides** – Support brain function and cognitive enhancement.
- **Immune-Modulating Peptides** – Strengthen the body's natural defenses.

- **Hormonal Peptides** – Balance endocrine function and optimize reproductive health.
- **Cosmetic Peptides** – Improve skin elasticity, collagen production, and hair growth.
- **Sexual Health Peptides** – Enhance libido, erectile function, and overall performance.

Introduction to Peptides

Peptides are short chains of amino acids connected by peptide bonds, usually made up of two to fifty amino acids. They are smaller than proteins but share a similar composition and act as essential building blocks in various biological processes. Peptides can occur naturally or be synthetically engineered, with applications in medicine, nutrition, and biotechnology. They are highly versatile molecules that often function as signaling molecules, hormones, enzyme regulators, or even structural components within cells and tissues. Their small size and specific biochemical functions make them invaluable in numerous fields.

In modern medicine, peptides have gained significant attention as therapeutic agents due to their high specificity, efficacy, and low toxicity. They can mimic the body's natural molecules, which allows for targeted treatments with fewer side effects compared to traditional drugs. Insulin, for example, is a well-known peptide hormone that is essential for the regulation of blood sugar levels in diabetes management. Other examples include glucagon-like peptide-1 (GLP-1) analogs used for diabetes and obesity, antimicrobial peptides for drug-resistant infections, and peptide-based drugs for cancer treatment. Peptides are also utilized in the development of vaccines, such as cancer immunotherapy and infectious disease prevention. Their ability to act precisely at cellular targets makes them a tool in the fight against complex diseases like neurodegenerative disorders and autoimmune conditions.

In the field of nutrition, peptides are increasingly recognized for their bioactive properties. These bioactive peptides are derived from proteins during digestion or through fermentation processes and exhibit various health benefits. For instance, certain peptides have antioxidant, anti-inflammatory, antimicrobial, and immune-boosting effects. They can also help lower blood pressure, improve gut health, and promote muscle recovery. As a result, bioactive peptides are incorporated into functional foods, dietary supplements, and sports nutrition products to support overall health and well-being.

Beyond medicine and nutrition, peptides have a wide range of applications in biotechnology, research, and cosmetic industries. In research, they are used as tools to study protein interactions, enzyme functions, and cellular mechanisms. Peptides also play a role in drug discovery and design, which enables the development of novel therapeutic agents. In cosmetics, peptides are incorporated into anti-aging products due to their ability to stimulate collagen production, improve skin elasticity, and reduce wrinkles.

The versatility of peptides stems from their ability to perform specific biological functions with precision. As advancements in peptide synthesis and delivery technologies continue, their potential applications continue to expand rapidly. From innovative medical therapies to health and nutrition and breakthroughs in biotechnology, peptides have become indispensable tools across various scientific and commercial fields. They help improve human health and advance science, which underscores their importance in the modern world.

Peptides are formed through a specific type of chemical reaction known as dehydration synthesis (or condensation reaction). This process involves the following key elements:

- Carboxyl Group (-COOH): The carboxyl group of one amino acid reacts with the amino group of another amino acid.
- Amino Group ($-NH_2$): The amino group of the second amino acid is involved in the reaction.
- Water Release: As a result of this reaction, a molecule of water (H_2O) is released.
- Covalent Amide Bond: The reaction creates a covalent bond known as a peptide bond (a specific type of amide bond), which links the two amino acids together.

This bond formation is critical to build peptides and proteins, which are essential for numerous biological functions.

Structural Levels of Peptides

Peptides exhibit different structural levels, each of which contributes to their overall function and stability. These levels include:

Primary Structure

The primary structure refers to the linear sequence of amino acids in a peptide chain. This sequence determines the basic function and characteristics of the peptide. The specific order of amino acids dictates how the peptide will fold and interact with other molecules. The primary structure is conventionally described from the N-terminus (the end with a free amino group) to the C-terminus (the end with a free carboxyl group).

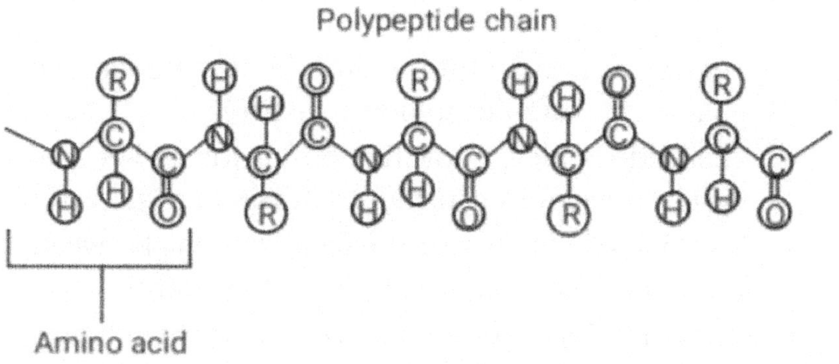

Fig 1: Primary structure

Secondary Structure

The secondary structure refers to localized fold patterns within the peptide chain.

- Alpha Helices: A coiled structure stabilized by hydrogen bonds between every fourth amino acid.
- Beta Sheets: A flat, sheet-like structure formed by hydrogen bonds between segments of the peptide chain that may be far apart in the primary sequence.

Secondary structures are mainly influenced by hydrogen bonds between the backbone atoms in the polypeptide chain.

Tertiary Structure

The tertiary structure refers to the overall three-dimensional shape of a single peptide or protein molecule. Factors include:

- Hydrogen Bonds: Interactions between polar side chains can stabilize folded structures.
- Disulfide Bridges: Covalent bonds formed between cysteine residues can stabilize protein structure.
- Van der Waals Forces: Weak attractions between nonpolar side chains contribute to stability.
- Hydrophobic Interactions: Nonpolar side chains tend to cluster away from water, which influences how the peptide folds.

Size Classification of Peptides

Peptides are classified based on their size, which is determined by the number of amino acids they contain. They include:

- Dipeptides: Composed of two amino acids linked by a peptide bond.
- Tripeptides: Consist of three amino acids.
- Oligopeptides: Contain between two and 20 amino acids. These are often involved in signaling and regulatory functions.
- Polypeptides: Comprise more than 20 amino acids. While some polypeptides fold into functional proteins, others remain as linear chains or require multiple polypeptide chains to form a complete protein.

Types of Peptides

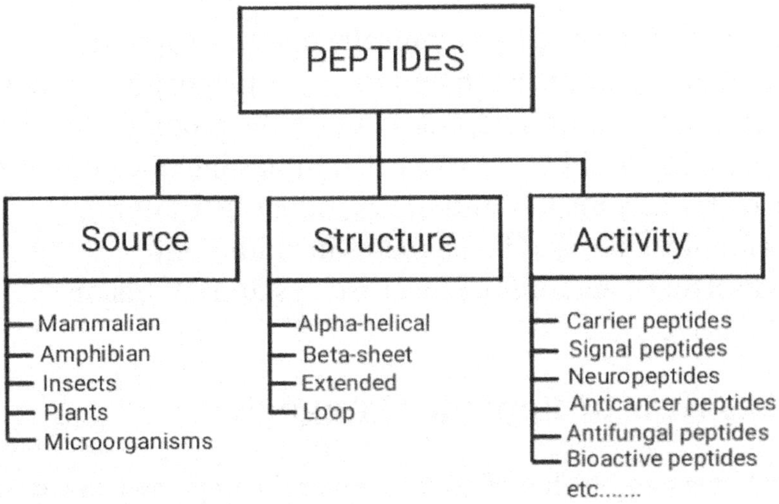

Fig 2: Types of peptides

Peptides can be classified based on their length and structure as:

- Oligopeptides: Chains that contain fewer than 20 amino acids.
- Polypeptides: Longer chains usually consist of 20 to 50 amino acids.
- Proteins: Larger structures formed from one or more polypeptide chains.

Peptides can also be categorized as natural, synthetic, or recombinant, depending on their origin and method of production. Natural peptides are produced by living organisms and play essential roles in biological functions such as hormone regulation and immune response. Examples include insulin (blood glucose regulation), oxytocin (labor and lactation), vasopressin (blood pressure control), and glucagon (glucose homeostasis).

Synthetic peptides are chemically manufactured in laboratories for research and therapeutic purposes. They often mimic natural peptides but can be modified for enhanced stability or activity. Examples include octreotide (used for acromegaly and neuroendocrine tumors), desmopressin (used for diabetes insipidus and bedwetting), and enfuvirtide (used as an HIV fusion inhibitor).

Overview of Peptide Categories

Peptides can be classified into several categories based on their applications:

- Therapeutic Peptides: Used in medical treatments, such as insulin for diabetes management or peptide hormones for growth regulation.
- Cosmetic Peptides: Incorporated into skin care products to promote collagen production and improve skin elasticity. Good examples are copper peptides (which support wound healing and collagen synthesis) and palmitoyl pentapeptide (which aids in reducing wrinkles and improving skin texture).
- Nutritional Peptides: Found in dietary supplements that support muscle growth and recovery.

Mechanisms of Action in the Human Body

The mechanisms of action of peptides in the human body are highly diverse based on their structure, target, and biological role. Generally, peptides interact with specific receptors, enzymes, or other molecules, which triggers physiological responses.

Receptor Binding and Signal Transduction

Many peptides act as signaling molecules, such as hormones or neurotransmitters, that bind to specific cell surface receptors (usually G-protein coupled receptors or receptor tyrosine kinases). Once they bind, they activate intracellular signaling pathways that regulate various cellular processes like metabolism, growth, and immune response.

- **Example**: Insulin, a peptide hormone, binds to the insulin receptor, which triggers pathways that facilitate glucose uptake and metabolism in cells.

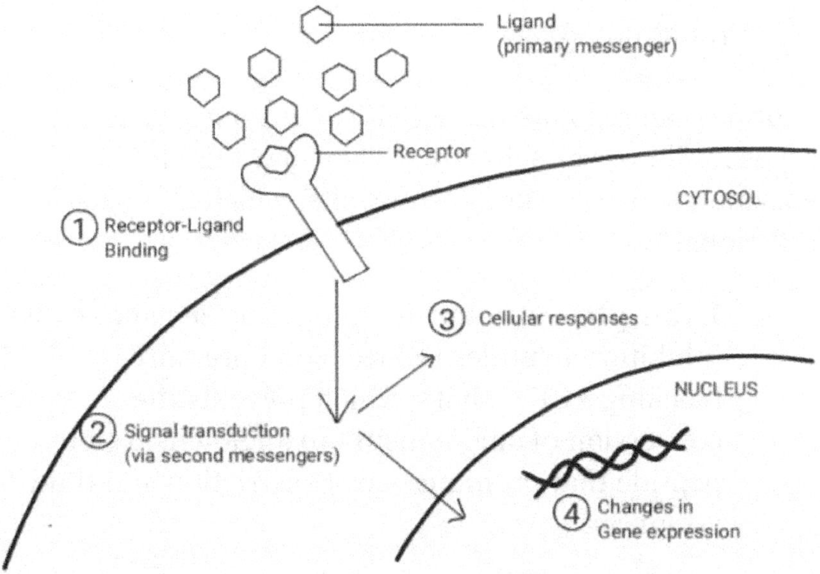

Fig 3: Receptor binding and signaling

Enzyme Inhibition or Activation

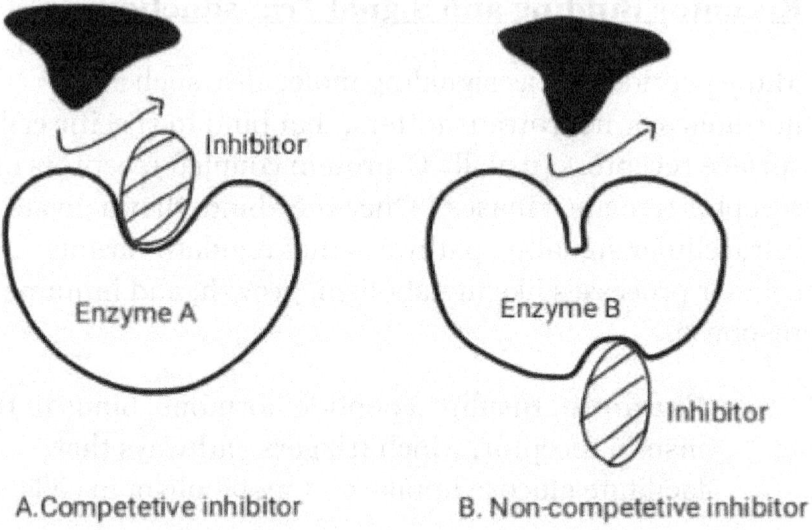

Fig 4: Inhibition types

Peptides can regulate the activity of enzymes when they act as inhibitors or activators. They may bind to the enzyme's active site or allosteric site, which alters its functionality.

- **Example**: Angiotensin-converting enzyme (ACE) inhibitory peptides reduce blood pressure by blocking ACE activity, which prevents the conversion of angiotensin I to angiotensin II, a peptide that promotes vasoconstriction and fluid retention.

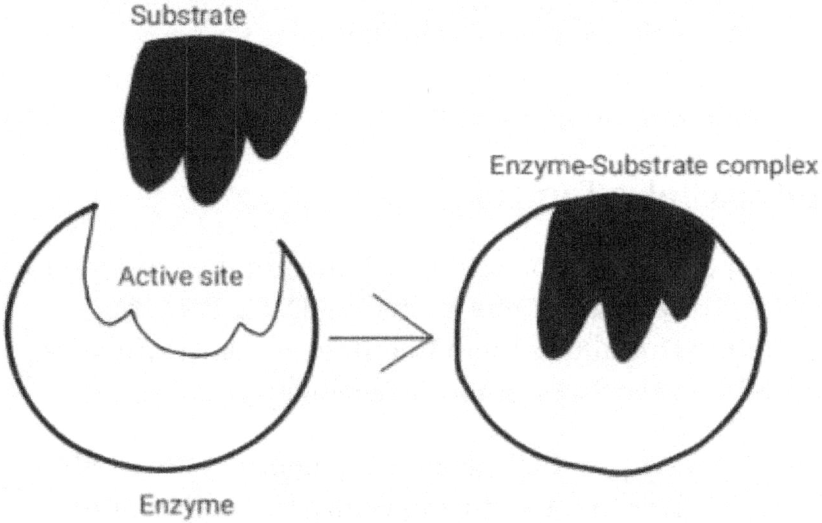

Fig 5: Enzyme-substrate interaction

Membrane Interaction and Permeabilization

Certain peptides, such as antimicrobial peptides (AMPs), interact directly with cell membranes. They can disrupt microbial membranes when they form pores or destabilize the lipid bilayer, which causes cell death. This is a critical defense mechanism against infections.

- **Example**: Defensins are AMPs that disrupt bacterial cell membranes, which causes lysis.

Immune System Modulation

Peptides can modulate immune system activity when they interact with immune cells. They may act as cytokines, chemokines, or immune enhancers. They regulate inflammation, immune surveillance, and tissue repair.

- **Example**: Thymosin alpha-1 enhances T-cell function and is used in therapies for immunodeficiency, viral infections, and cancer immunotherapy.

Intracellular Targets

Some peptides can penetrate cell membranes and interact with intracellular targets, including DNA, RNA, or proteins. This allows them to influence gene expression, protein synthesis, or other intracellular processes.

- **Example**: Cell-penetrating peptides are used to deliver therapeutic molecules like siRNA or drugs into cells.

Neurotransmitter Function

Neuroactive peptides, such as substance P and endorphins, act as neurotransmitters or neuromodulators in the nervous system. They bind to receptors in the brain and peripheral nervous system, which influences pain perception, mood, and behavior.

- **Example**: Endorphins bind to opioid receptors, which produce pain relief and euphoria.

Antioxidant and Anti-Inflammatory Effects

Certain peptides neutralize free radicals or inhibit pro-inflammatory mediators, which protect cells and tissues from oxidative stress and inflammation.

- **Example**: Bioactive peptides derived from food proteins (e.g., casein hydrolysates) scavenge free radicals, which reduces oxidative damage.

Stimulate Collagen Production and Tissue Repair

Peptides involved in wound healing and skin repair can stimulate collagen synthesis or promote angiogenesis. These actions are often exploited in cosmetic and therapeutic products.

- **Example**: Matrixyl peptides in skin care stimulate fibroblasts to produce collagen, which improves skin elasticity and reduces wrinkles.

Hormonal Regulation

Peptides often function as hormones that regulate physiological processes. These hormones act as messengers to coordinate endocrine functions, such as metabolism, growth, and reproduction.

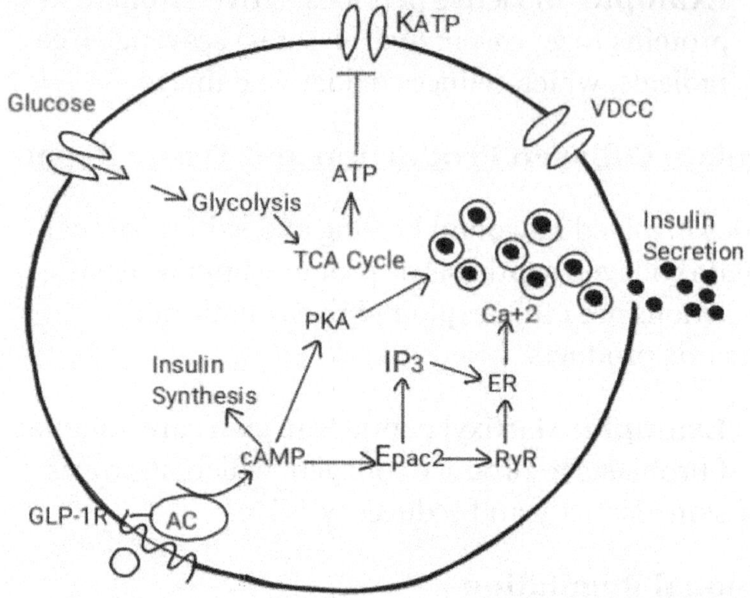

Fig 6: GLP-1 stimulates insulin release

- **Example**: GLP-1 stimulates insulin secretion, slows gastric emptying, and suppresses glucagon release, which collectively helps regulate blood glucose levels.

Gene Expression Modulation

Some therapeutic peptides are designed to bind to specific DNA or RNA sequences, which influences gene expression. This mechanism is being explored in gene therapy and cancer treatment.

- **Example**: Peptides used in epigenetic therapy modify chromatin structure and gene transcription.

Historical Context and Discovery of Peptides

Our knowledge of peptides has evolved over centuries, with significant milestones in both scientific discovery and technological innovation. The historical context of peptides showcases how advances in chemistry, biology, and medicine have progressively uncovered their structures, functions, and applications.

Early Observations (18th-19th Century)

Foundations in Protein Chemistry: In the late 18th century, scientists like Antoine Fourcroy and Jöns Jacob Berzelius studied proteins and their role in living organisms. Although peptides were not yet distinguished, these early studies laid the groundwork for our modern knowledge of proteins as macromolecules essential to life.

Proteins were first recognized as complex molecules composed of smaller subunits, but their exact composition was unknown.

Identification of Amino Acids: Louis-Nicolas Vauquelin and Pierre Jean Robiquet, two French chemists, discovered asparagine, the first amino acid, in 1806. During the 19th century, additional amino acids were identified, including glycine, leucine, and tyrosine.

By the late 19th century, Emil Fischer, a German chemist, made critical contributions when he demonstrated that proteins are composed of amino acids linked by peptide bonds. Fischer's work earned him the Nobel Prize in Chemistry in 1902 and introduced the term "peptide."

Peptide Chemistry in the Early 20th Century

Elucidation of Peptide Bonds: Emil Fischer and Franz Hofmeister provided the first insights into peptide bonds—the chemical links between amino acids. They synthesized small peptides in the laboratory and demonstrated that these molecules could be artificially constructed.

Fischer's work confirmed that peptides were intermediate structures between free amino acids and larger proteins.

Hormonal Peptides: In 1921, Frederick Banting and Charles Best discovered insulin, a peptide hormone critical for the regulation of blood glucose levels. Insulin was one of the first peptides identified with a specific physiological role. This revolutionized diabetes treatment and advanced the field of endocrinology.

Oxytocin and vasopressin, two other key peptide hormones, were identified in the mid-20th century, which further highlights the importance of peptides in the regulation of physiological processes.

Advancements in Peptide Synthesis (1930s–1960s)

Chemical Synthesis of Peptides: Robert Bruce Merrifield, an American biochemist, developed the solid-phase peptide synthesis technique in 1963, which allowed for the efficient and automated production of peptides. This work earned Merrifield the Nobel Prize in Chemistry in 1984.

Structural Characterization: Advances in techniques such as x-ray crystallography and nuclear magnetic resonance spectroscopy in the mid-20th century allowed for detailed structural studies of peptides. These tools provided insights into their three-dimensional structure and biological interactions.

Peptides in Biotechnology and Medicine (1970s–Present)

Therapeutic Peptides: The discovery of synthetic insulin in the 1970s marked a major milestone in peptide-based therapies. It demonstrated the potential of peptides to replace or supplement natural hormones in disease management.

Over the decades, other therapeutic peptides were developed, such as calcitonin for osteoporosis, GLP-1 agonists for diabetes, and AMPs for infections.

Peptide Vaccines: Peptides began to be explored in vaccine development due to their ability to stimulate immune responses. In modern medicine, peptide-based vaccines have been developed for cancer and infectious diseases.

Peptides in Diagnostics and Research: Peptides play a vital role as biomarkers and research tools. Radioactive and fluorescently labeled peptides are used in diagnostic imaging, while peptide fragments are employed to study protein function and cellular signaling.

Current Era and Future Directions

Peptide Therapeutics Boom: The pharmaceutical industry has seen an explosion in peptide-based drug development, which targets diseases such as cancer, autoimmune disorders, and neurodegenerative conditions.

Peptides in Biotechnology: Peptides are widely used in biotechnology, from drug development to synthetic biology. Techniques like CRISPR-Cas9, for instance, leverage RNA-guided systems to edit genes.

Peptides in Nutrition and Cosmetics: Bioactive peptides derived from food proteins are incorporated into functional foods and supplements for health benefits like improved digestion, cardiovascular health, and immune support. In cosmetics, peptides are used to stimulate collagen production and improve skin health.

Applications of Peptides in Modern Science and Medicine

Peptides are increasingly utilized in diverse scientific and medical applications.

- **Drug Development:** Many new drugs are based on peptide structures due to their specificity and low toxicity.
- **Cancer Therapy:** Targeted peptide therapies attack cancer cells, which spares healthy tissues.
- **Vaccines:** Peptide-based vaccines are designed to elicit immune responses against specific pathogens.
- **Tissue Engineering:** Peptides are used to create scaffolds that support cell growth and tissue regeneration.

Chapter 1: Peptides and Their Role in Fat Loss

In recent years, the use of peptides in fat metabolism has gained significant attention, particularly in the management of obesity and metabolic disorders. They have emerged as a significant focus in weight loss strategies due to their multifaceted roles in fat metabolism, appetite regulation, and muscle preservation.

Mechanism of Peptides in Fat Metabolism

Peptides play a critical role in the regulation of fat metabolism through their interactions with hormonal pathways and signaling systems. The key mechanisms include:

- Lipolysis Activation: Many peptides stimulate the breakdown of triglycerides stored in fat cells, a process known as lipolysis.
- Improved Insulin Sensitivity: Some peptides modulate insulin activity, which prevents excessive fat storage. For example, GLP-1 receptor agonists improve insulin secretion and reduce insulin resistance, which helps to maintain stable blood glucose levels.
- Boosted Basal Metabolic Rate: Peptides such as growth hormone (GH) secretagogues increase energy expenditure. They promote lean muscle mass and reduce fat accumulation.
- Appetite Regulation: Certain peptides influence the hypothalamus to regulate hunger and satiety.

Popular Peptides Used for Fat Loss

Several peptides are commonly used in clinical and therapeutic settings to support fat loss. Each has a unique mechanism of action.

GLP-1 Receptor Agonists

Some of the most common GLP-1 receptor agonists are semaglutide and liraglutide.

Structure and Property

GLP-1 receptor agonists are synthetic peptides that mimic the incretin hormone GLP-1. These peptides are modified to resist enzymatic degradation by dipeptidyl peptidase-4 (DPP-4), which prolongs their half-life in the bloodstream.

Mechanism of Action

GLP-1 agonists enhance insulin secretion in a glucose-dependent manner, inhibit glucagon release, and delay gastric emptying. They act on the hypothalamus to regulate appetite and promote satiety, which reduces caloric intake.

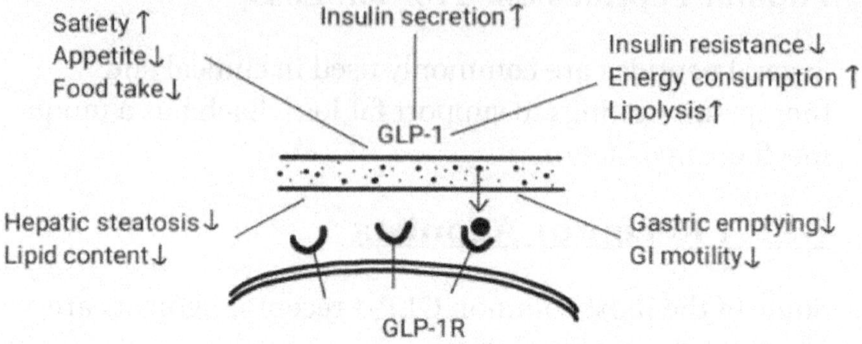

Fig 7: Mechanism of action of GLP-1

Clinical Implications:

- Help manage obesity and Type 2 diabetes.
- Improve glycemic control and aid in weight loss.
- Reduce cardiovascular risks in high-risk populations.

Administration and Nursing Considerations

- Emphasize proper injection technique, including site rotation and preparation, to minimize infection risk.
- Ensure patients adhere to storage requirements (typically refrigeration for some formulations) and use proper disposal protocols for used needles, following manufacturer guidelines.
- Timing considerations are critical. Patients should administer semaglutide on a consistent weekly schedule and be educated on missed dose protocols as well as potential food interactions.

Ongoing monitoring should include:

- Regularly track weight changes and blood glucose levels.
- Monitor for gastrointestinal symptoms and evaluate patient compliance with therapy.

Side Effects

- Common: Nausea, vomiting, diarrhea, and abdominal pain.
- Rare: Pancreatitis or gallbladder disorders.

Patients need to be started with a low dose that is gradually increased to improve tolerance. Encourage hydration and dietary adjustments to manage gastrointestinal symptoms.

CJC-1295 and Ipamorelin

Structure and Property

CJC-1295 is a synthetic analog of growth hormone-releasing hormone (GHRH) with added modifications to extend its half-life (seven to eight days). Ipamorelin is a selective GH secretagogue that mimics ghrelin's effects. It has a short half-life, which makes it ideal for controlled doses.

Mechanism of Action

These peptides stimulate the pituitary gland to release GH. Elevated GH levels enhance lipolysis and promote fat breakdown. They also preserve lean muscle mass and improve tissue repair and metabolic function.

Clinical Implications

- Used in fitness and medical settings to improve body composition.
- Help reduce visceral fat and improve energy levels.
- May support muscle recovery in patients in rehabilitation.

Administration and Nursing Considerations

Dosing usually involves subcutaneous injections, with specific regimens based on individual patient needs and treatment goals. Common dosing may range from one to two milligrams per week, divided into multiple doses.

CJC-1295 that is administered at night may optimize GH release due to its natural pulsing pattern during sleep. Timing can also be adjusted based on individual schedules and responses.

Side Effects

- Common: Injection site reactions (e.g., redness, swelling).
- Rare: Headaches, water retention, or joint pain.

Ensure proper injection technique to minimize local reactions. Monitor for excessive fluid retention or signs of carpal tunnel syndrome.

Tesamorelin

Tesamorelin is a synthetic analog of GHRH designed to stimulate GH secretion. It has a high specificity for GHRH receptors and minimizes off-target effects.

Mechanism of Action

Tesamorelin acts on the hypothalamus and pituitary gland to increase GH release. This causes enhanced lipolysis, which especially targets visceral fat stores. It also improves insulin sensitivity.

Clinical Implications

- Approved for the reduction of abdominal fat in patients with HIV-associated lipodystrophy.
- Has potential applications in general visceral fat reduction and metabolic syndrome.
- May improve patient confidence and quality of life through the reduction of fat accumulation.

Administration and Nursing Considerations

Tesamorelin is injected subcutaneously into the abdomen. The navel area must be avoided. Rotation of the injection site is critical to prevent localized irritation or lipodystrophy. Tesamorelin should be administered at the same time each day, preferably at night, to mimic the natural circadian rhythm of GH secretion.

Tesamorelin is administered as a subcutaneous injection of 2 mg once daily. For the EGRIFTA SV formulation, the reconstituted solution contains 1.4 mg per 0.35 mL, and requires appropriate dosage adjustments as per the manufacturer guidelines.

Side Effects

- Common: Mild edema, muscle pain, and injection site reactions.

- Rare: Hyperglycemia or worsened diabetes in some patients.

Regulation: Regularly monitor blood glucose levels, particularly in patients with pre-existent diabetes or impaired glucose tolerance.

AOD-9604

Structure and Property

AOD-9604 is a synthetic analog of a fragment of the human GH molecule, specifically amino acids 176–191, which has been studied for its potential role in fat metabolism. This makes it highly specific for fat metabolism and does not affect blood sugar levels.

Mechanism of Action

AOD-9604 stimulates lipolysis and inhibits lipogenesis. It directly acts on adipose tissues. It does not influence insulin-like growth factor (IGF-1) levels or induce general growth effects, which makes it safer for targeted fat loss.

Clinical Implications

- Used to reduce stubborn fat deposits, particularly in overweight and obese individuals.
- May benefit patients who cannot tolerate systemic metabolic changes caused by other peptides.
- Non-anabolic, which makes it a safer choice for broader populations.

Administration and Nursing Considerations

When they administer AOD-9604, nurses should be aware of several important considerations. AOD-9604 is usually administered via subcutaneous injection. Nurses should ensure proper technique and hygiene to minimize infection risk. The peptide should be stored in a cool, dry place, ideally at temperatures between 2°C and 8°C (36°F to 46°F). Avoid exposure to light and moisture to maintain stability.

The standard dosage for AOD-9604 is 300 mcg (micrograms) per day. This is generally taken in the morning, approximately 30 minutes before meals, for optimal results. It is administered via subcutaneous injection, ideally into fatty areas such as the abdomen.

Side Effects

- Common: Mild headaches or localized discomfort at injection sites.
- Rare: Allergic reactions or gastrointestinal upset.

Rotate injection sites to prevent tissue irritation. Monitor for any signs of hypersensitivity or adverse reactions.

Amylin Analogs (e.g., Pramlintide)

Structure and Property

Pramlintide is a synthetic version of amylin, a hormone co-secreted with insulin by pancreatic beta cells. It is structurally stable, which ensures longer activity compared to endogenous amylin.

Mechanism of Action

Pramlintide slows gastric emptying and suppresses glucagon release postprandially. It promotes satiety because it acts on the brain's centers for appetite regulation, which reduces meal sizes and caloric intake.

Clinical Implications

- Approved for use in diabetes management to complement insulin therapy.
- Effectively reduces appetite and supports weight loss in overweight patients.

Side Effects

- Common: Nausea, hypoglycemia (when combined with insulin).
- Rare: Severe hypoglycemia or allergic reactions.

Titrate doses cautiously, particularly in diabetic patients, to avoid hypoglycemia. Encourage small, frequent meals to improve tolerance.

Role of Growth Hormone in Fat Reduction

GH is a key player in fat metabolism. It works through several mechanisms to promote fat loss.

- Lipolysis Enhancement: GH stimulates hormone-sensitive lipase, an enzyme that breaks down stored triglycerides in adipose tissue.
- Muscle Preservation: Because it encourages protein synthesis, GH preserves lean muscle mass, which is essential to maintain a higher basal metabolic rate.

- Insulin Regulation: GH can reduce insulin sensitivity in some cases, alter fat storage, and influence glucose metabolism.

Peptides like CJC-1295 and Ipamorelin are designed to mimic the body's natural GH release, which provides therapeutic benefits for fat loss. Nurses should understand the physiological effects of GH to monitor patients effectively and address any adverse reactions.

Effects of Peptides on Appetite and Satiety

The regulation of appetite and satiety is a critical aspect of peptide therapy for weight loss. Several peptides target the brain's hunger centers, particularly in the hypothalamus.

- **GLP-1 Receptor Agonists:** These peptides slow gastric emptying, which creates a sensation of fullness and reduces overall calorie intake. Patients often report significant appetite suppression, which helps in long-term weight management.
- **Amylin Analogs (e.g., Pramlintide):** Amylin works alongside insulin to slow gastric emptying and regulate post-meal glucose levels. Because they mimic amylin, peptides like Pramlintide enhance satiety but do not significantly reduce meal sizes.
- **Leptin and Ghrelin Modulation**: Peptides that influence leptin (the satiety hormone) and ghrelin (the hunger hormone) further help regulate eating behavior.

Risks and Side Effects Associated with Fat Loss Peptides

Although peptides provide benefits, they are not without risks. Nurses must be aware of potential side effects and educate patients on safe usage.

- Hormonal Imbalance: Overstimulation of hormone production can lead to imbalances that may affect metabolism and overall health.
- Local Reactions at the Injection Site: Injectable peptides may result in injection site discomfort, edema, or redness.
- Long-Term Effects: The long-term safety profile of many weight-loss peptides is still under investigation, which necessitates caution and further research before widespread use.

Long-Term Risks

Some peptides may influence glucose metabolism, which causes hypoglycemia in susceptible individuals. There are concerns about the potential link between long-term peptide use and tumor growth due to their impact on cell proliferation. Misuse of peptides in nonmedical settings can lead to unregulated dosages and unsafe practices.

Contraindications

Peptides are not recommended for individuals with a history of certain cancers or endocrine disorders.

Chapter 2: Peptides to Build Muscle

Peptides have gained significant popularity in the fitness and bodybuilding communities due to their ability to enhance muscle growth, promote fat loss, and improve recovery times. These molecules, composed of short chains of amino acids, can regulate various biological processes because they mimic or influence the body's natural signaling pathways. In the context of fitness and muscle-building, peptides stimulate mechanisms such as GH secretion, muscle protein synthesis, and tissue repair, which makes them a valuable tool for athletes and bodybuilders who want to optimize their physical performance and recovery.

Peptides especially promote muscle growth because they can target specific pathways that regulate anabolic processes, muscle repair, and recovery. Many of these peptides directly stimulate growth factors, such as GH and IGF-1, or enhance cellular repair mechanisms.

- **IGF-1**: This factor promotes protein synthesis, a process that repairs and builds muscle tissue, especially after exercise. This repair is critical for muscle hypertrophy (an increase in muscle size) as it ensures that muscle protein synthesis happens faster than muscle protein breakdown.
- **BPC-157**: This synthetic peptide, derived from a protein found in gastric juice, supports tissue repair and stimulates angiogenesis (the growth of new blood vessels). Because it improves blood supply to damaged tissues, it helps with healing and recovery.

- **IGF-1 LR3**: It extends the half-life of IGF-1 and improves protein synthesis and cellular growth, but its role in muscle recovery and hypertrophy requires further clinical validation.

These peptides improve communication between cells and speed up the repair and rebuilding of muscle fibers after physical activity. They essentially enhance the body's natural recovery mechanisms and make them a valuable tool in muscle rehabilitation and growth.

Popular Peptides for Muscle Growth

Peptides are increasingly recognized for their role in muscle growth, recovery, and overall physical health.

BPC-157

BPC-157 is a synthetic peptide that promotes the healing of joints, tendons, and muscles. It accelerates the activity of fibroblasts and stimulates collagen production. Collagen is a key protein needed for the strength and structure of connective tissues.

This peptide is particularly helpful for patients who have overuse injuries, such as tendonitis or ligament strains, as well as exercise-induced damage. Its ability to speed up tissue repair makes it an attractive option for athletes or active individuals who need to recover quickly. Nurses may encounter patients who use BPC-157 to manage chronic joint pain or aid in injury recovery.

IGF-1 LR3

IGF-1 LR3 is a modified version of IGF-1. It helps increase muscle growth by stimulating protein synthesis, which is essential for muscle repair. However, its direct role in reducing muscle protein breakdown remains inconclusive in human studies. This modified version has a longer effect than natural IGF-1, which makes IGF-1 LR3 more efficient.

IGF-1 LR3 is often used by individuals who want to build lean muscle mass or recover from intense physical activity. It's particularly beneficial for patients in rehabilitation after injury or surgery, as it can help rebuild muscle and prevent loss of strength.

The usual BPC-157 dosage ranges from 200 to 1,000 micrograms, but the appropriate dosage can vary for each patient based on their medical history and treatment needs. Initial dosages usually range from 250 to 500 mcg per day. This may be gradually increased to 500 to 750 mcg daily, split into two to three injections.

Injection dosage is usually based on body weight and ranges from 150 to 375 mcg twice daily. A suggested dosage is to inject 0.15 mL (300 mcg) subcutaneously daily for 30 days. Oral doses usually range from 100 to 500 mcg, taken one to two times daily for injury recovery, inflammation management, and general healing.

A basic dose is 2.5 to 3.75 micrograms/kilogram of body weight twice a day. For a 60-kg person, this would be 150 to 225 mcg. For a 70-kg person, this would be 175 to 260 mcg.

Some practitioners suggest cycling, with a 6- to 12-week usage period followed by a four- to eight-week break between cycles. After an eight-week treatment period, it's common to cycle off BPC-157 for eight to ten weeks before potentially starting another cycle.

CJC-1295 and Ipamorelin (Combination)

These two peptides are often used together because of their complementary effects on GH production. CJC-1295 stimulates the release of GH from the pituitary gland, while Ipamorelin also promotes GH release with minimal impact on cortisol and prolactin levels, reducing potential stress-related effects.

This combination is critical for its ability to improve muscle recovery, support fat loss, boost energy levels, and promote lean muscle growth. The dual action makes it effective and minimizes side effects. Nurses may encounter patients who use this combination to manage age-related muscle loss, improve recovery from injuries, or enhance athletic performance.

A combined dosage might be 1 mg of CJC-1295 with 100 mcg of Ipamorelin, administered subcutaneously once daily or several times a week, based on individual needs. Another common dosage is 100 to 300 micrograms (mcg) of CJC-1295/Ipamorelin per day in single or divided doses.

Ibutamoren (MK-677)

Unlike other peptides that are injected, Ibutamoren is taken orally. It stimulates the release of both GH and IGF-1, which play key roles in muscle growth, fat loss, and recovery. One unique feature of Ibutamoren is its ability to maintain steady levels of these hormones for an extended period, which contributes to sustained benefits.

Ibutamoren is particularly good for patients who want the benefits of increased GH and IGF-1 without injections. In addition to its impact on muscle growth and fat reduction, it also improves sleep quality. Nurses might see this peptide used by patients who have muscle-wasting conditions, who want to enhance performance, or who seek to manage age-related declines in hormone levels.

Ibutamoren is commonly available in strengths of 10 mg and 25 mg, with 25 mg being the most frequently used dosage for muscle growth and fat loss. A dosage of 25 mg taken daily is considered optimal for muscle growth and fat loss. It should be taken at the same time each day. A typical dose for men is 25 mg at night.

Synergistic Effects of Peptides and Exercise

Peptides are most effective when used alongside regular exercise, particularly resistance training. Exercise naturally stimulates the release of GH, and peptides amplify this process, which enhances muscle growth and recovery. For nurses who work with patients who use peptides, knowledge of how these substances interact with exercise can help guide conversations about timing, usage, and maximum benefits.

- **Natural GH Release**: Resistance training naturally triggers the release of GH, which supports muscle growth, tissue repair, and fat metabolism. When peptides such as IGF-1 LR3 are used in combination with exercise, they enhance these effects. IGF-1 LR3 promotes protein synthesis, but its effects on long-term muscle hypertrophy in humans remain under investigation. This means that after strength training, muscle gains can be more substantial when peptides are included as part of the regimen.

- **Inflammation Reduction**: Intense exercise often causes inflammation in the muscles and joints, which can cause soreness and slow recovery. Certain peptides, such as BPC-157, have anti-inflammatory properties that help reduce exercise-induced inflammation. This allows individuals to recover faster and train more frequently, which is critical to build strength and endurance over time.

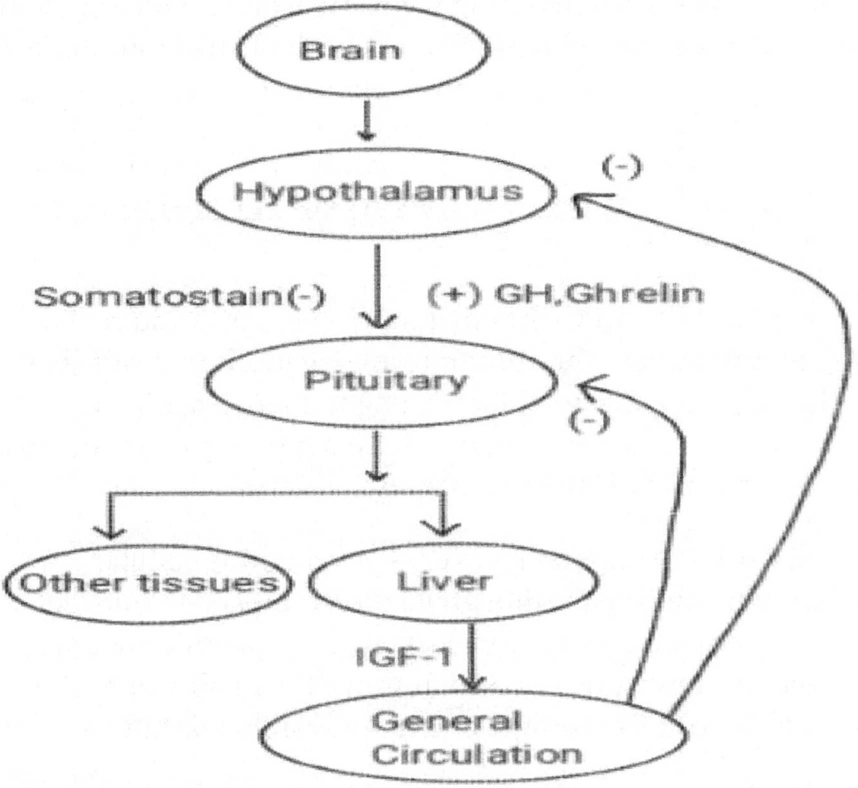

Fig 8: Natural GH release

The timing of peptide administration is critical to maximize effects. Research suggests that peptides taken around exercise sessions, either shortly before or after training, can prolong the body's anabolic (muscle-building) state.

- **CJC-1295 and Ipamorelin:** These GH-releasing peptides are particularly effective when administered near workouts. Taken before or after training, they help maintain elevated GH levels for an extended period, which promotes muscle repair and growth during recovery. Nurses who work with patients who use these peptides can emphasize the importance of a consistent schedule to achieve the best results.

Role of Peptides in Injury Recovery and Muscle Repair

Peptides like BPC-157 enhance tissue repair and reduce inflammation. They promote angiogenesis and collagen production, essential for healing tendons, ligaments, and muscles. Athletes often use these peptides to recover from strains or tears more efficiently.

IGF-1 LR3 supports recovery by promoting cellular growth and repair, though its direct impact on nutrient transport remains inconclusive. These peptides not only reduce downtime but also improve the quality of healing, which ensures stronger and more resilient tissues.

Risks, Legal Status, and Ethical Considerations of Peptides

Peptides have gained attention for their potential to promote muscle growth, recovery, and injury repair. However, nurses must be aware of the associated risks, legal limitations, and ethical concerns to guide patients appropriately.

Risks and Potential Side Effects

Although these peptides are generally well-tolerated, they are not without risks. Patients who use peptides should be closely monitored for adverse effects, which may include:

- **Joint Pain**: Some peptides can cause discomfort in joints, particularly during the initial stages of use. This can be due to changes in tissue repair or fluid retention.
- **Water Retention**: Peptides that influence GH levels, such as CJC-1295 and Ibutamoren, can cause fluid retention, particularly in individuals who are prone to edema or metabolic imbalances.
- **Adverse Immune Reactions:** In rare cases, peptides can trigger immune responses, including localized irritation at injection sites or systemic reactions like rashes or fatigue.
- **Hormonal Imbalances:** Improper use of peptides that affect GH or IGF-1 levels may result in unwanted hormonal effects, such as insulin resistance or elevated blood sugar levels. Nurses should educate patients about these risks and emphasize the importance of proper dosing and medical supervision.

Legal Status of Peptides

Many peptides, including BPC-157 and IGF-1 LR3, are not FDA-approved for human use outside of specific research settings. They are usually available only for research purposes or under experimental protocols. This means that patients using these peptides may access them through unregulated channels, which carries risks of contamination, inaccurate dosing, or counterfeit products.

Some peptides, such as GLP-1 receptor agonists, can be legally prescribed for approved medical conditions, but others, like BPC-157 and IGF-1 LR3, are not approved for off-label human use. Nurses should remind patients that peptides obtained from unverified sources, such as online vendors, pose significant safety risks.

Ethical Considerations in Sports and Fitness

The use of peptides in sports is a contentious issue. Organizations like the World Anti-Doping Agency have banned many peptides, including IGF-1 derivatives, because they can enhance performance. Athletes who use these substances risk disqualification, fines, and damage to their reputations.

From an ethical standpoint, the use of peptides to gain an unfair advantage in competitive sports undermines the principles of fair play. Nurses who work with athletes should counsel them on the ethical implications of banned substances and explore alternative legal options for recovery and performance improvement.

The Role of Nurses

Nurses guide patients through the risks, legal implications, and ethical considerations of peptide use.

- **Patient Education**: Educate patients about the potential side effects of peptides. Emphasize that they should be obtained through legitimate medical channels. Explain that unregulated products carry significant risks, including contamination and incorrect dosing.
- **Legal Awareness**: Ensure patients understand the legal status of the peptides they want to use.

For athletes, discuss the consequences of violations of anti-doping regulations.

- **Ethics**: For patients in competitive sports, explore the ethical concerns associated with banned peptides. Nurses can encourage patients to focus on natural methods of recovery and performance enhancement, such as nutrition, physical therapy, and proper training techniques.
- **Monitor and Support**: For patients who choose to use peptides under medical supervision, nurses can monitor for side effects, track progress, and provide support to ensure safe and effective use.

Comparison with Anabolic Steroids

Unlike anabolic steroids, which include synthetic derivatives of testosterone, some peptides stimulate natural hormone release, while others may still exert hormone-like effects. This mechanism reduces the risk of hormonal imbalances and side effects like liver damage and cardiovascular issues. However, peptides often take longer to show results compared to steroids, which deliver immediate but often unsustainable gains.

Peptides are also more targeted, which influences specific pathways such as GH release or collagen synthesis. This makes them suitable for injury recovery and long-term muscle maintenance. Steroids, on the other hand, have broader effects and often cause unintended consequences, such as aggression or suppressed natural hormone production.

Chapter 3: Peptides for Longevity

Peptides are a promising tool in the field of longevity research, with their ability to modulate biological processes that influence aging and overall health. Aging is a complex process characterized by a gradual decline in cellular function, tissue repair, and immune efficiency. Peptides can interact with specific receptors in the body to regulate pathways associated with aging, repair, and rejuvenation. Their potential to enhance health span (the period of life spent in good health) and possibly extend life span makes them a focus in modern medicine and longevity science.

Role of Peptides that Lengthen Telomeres (e.g., Epitalon)

Telomeres are repetitive nucleotide sequences located at the termini of chromosomes. They serve as protective caps that maintain genomic stability. Each time a cell divides, its telomeres shorten, which eventually causes cellular senescence or apoptosis when they become critically short. This progressive shortening is a hallmark of aging and contributes to the decline in tissue function over time.

Epitalon, a synthetic tetrapeptide (Ala-Glu-Asp-Gly), is based on a naturally occurring pineal gland peptide and has garnered attention for its potential anti-aging properties. One of its primary mechanisms is the activation of telomerase, an enzyme that adds telomeric repeats to the ends of chromosomes, which counteracts telomere shortening. In vitro studies have demonstrated that Epitalon induces telomerase activity and elongates telomeres in human somatic cells.

Specifically, research on human fetal fibroblast cultures suggested that Epitalon treatment may influence the expression of the catalytic subunit of telomerase. This may potentially increase enzymatic activity and affect telomere length. This suggests that Epitalon can reactivate the telomerase gene in somatic cells, potentially extend their life span, and enhance overall organismal longevity.

Beyond its effects on telomeres, Epitalon has been shown to influence various physiological processes associated with aging. Animal studies indicate that Epitalon can normalize circadian rhythms because it regulates melatonin secretion, a hormone pivotal in sleep-wake cycles and overall circadian regulation. In aging rats, Epitalon treatment restored the daily rhythm of melatonin production. It aligned it more closely with patterns observed in younger animals. This normalization of circadian rhythms is critical, as disruptions are linked to various age-related disorders.

Epitalon appears to modulate the immune system. Research in aging mice demonstrated that Epitalon reduced the incidence of chromosomal aberrations, which suggests a protective effect on genomic integrity. Additionally, studies have shown that Epitalon can enhance the activity of antioxidant enzymes, such as superoxide dismutase and glutathione peroxidase, which combat oxidative stress and are significant contributors to cellular aging.

In elderly patients, preliminary studies have suggested that Epitalon administration may be associated with changes in telomere length in blood cells, but further research is needed to confirm its potential role in cellular rejuvenation. Some preliminary studies have suggested that Epitalon treatment may influence markers associated with aging, but conclusive long-term studies on overall mortality and age-related disease incidence are lacking.

Peptides Target Oxidative Stress and Inflammation

Oxidative stress arises when the generation of reactive oxygen species (ROS) surpasses the body's antioxidant defenses, which causes cellular damage. This imbalance is a significant contributor to aging and the development of chronic diseases. Peptides like BPC-157 and thymosin beta-4 (TB4) have demonstrated efficacy in the fight against oxidative stress and inflammation.

Tissue Protection and Healing

BPC-157 safeguards tissues from oxidative damage and facilitates cellular recovery. Studies have shown that BPC-157 can counteract oxidative stress and maintain the function of the nitric oxide system, which is critical for vascular health.

Inflammation Reduction and Cellular Protection

TB4 and its fragments play a pivotal role in the diminishment of inflammation. They shield cells from oxidative injury because they modulate immune responses. Research indicates that TB4 prevents oxidative stress, inflammation, and fibrosis in various tissues, which highlights its therapeutic potential.

Chronic inflammation, often termed "inflammaging," is a fundamental factor in many age-related conditions. Peptides like BPC-157 and TB4 modulate inflammatory pathways. They target cytokines such as TNF-α, IL-1β, and IL-6. Because they regulate these pro-inflammatory molecules, these peptides help reduce tissue degradation and restore physiological balance.

Peptides Promote Cellular Repair and Regeneration

Peptide therapy represents a novel approach in the field of regenerative medicine, with its most profound impact seen in cellular repair and tissue regeneration. Peptides are short chains of amino acids that can act as signaling molecules, which directly influence processes essential for the maintenance and restoration of tissue integrity. They enhance the body's natural repair mechanisms and provide resilience against the cumulative damage associated with aging.

BPC-157

BPC-157 is a synthetic peptide composed of 15 amino acids derived from a protein found in gastric juice. It is renowned for its remarkable healing properties and tissue regeneration effects.

Mechanisms of Action

- **Promotion of Accelerated Healing**: BPC-157 stimulates the production of growth factors and promotes angiogenesis (the formation of new blood vessels), which is critical for wound healing and tissue repair.

- **Tissue Regeneration**: It enhances the expression of GH receptors in various cells and aids in the regeneration of tendons, muscles, ligaments, and bones.

- **Anti-Inflammatory Properties**: It exhibits potent anti-inflammatory effects and helps to reduce inflammation and associated tissue damage.

- **Improved Blood Flow**: Because it increases blood flow to specific areas, BPC-157 ensures adequate oxygen and nutrient supply essential for repair processes.

- **Tissue Repair and Angiogenesis**: BPC-157 is renowned for its exceptional ability to support tissue repair. Because it promotes angiogenesis or the formation of new blood vessels, BPC-157 ensures that damaged tissues, such as ligaments, muscles, and other connective structures, receive adequate oxygen and nutrients to accelerate the healing process. This peptide facilitates rapid recovery because it improves vascularization in injury sites, which reduces recovery time.

- **Cell Survival and Fibroblast Migration**: Under conditions of stress, such as injury or inflammation, fibroblasts play a critical role in tissue repair. They produce collagen and extracellular matrix components. BPC-157 enhances the survival and migration of these fibroblasts, which ensures sustained tissue regeneration and long-term functional recovery. These actions make BPC-157 indispensable in the treatment of injuries and degenerative conditions.

Thymosin Beta-4 (TB4)

- **Cytoskeletal Repair:** Thymosin beta-4 contributes to the repair of the cytoskeleton, which provides structural support and mobility to cells. Because it regulates actin, a protein vital for cytoskeletal integrity, TB4 promotes cellular processes like migration, division, and repair.

- **Heals Cardiac and Nervous Tissues:** TB4 has shown remarkable efficacy in the repair of cardiac tissue after ischemic damage. It supports the regeneration of nervous tissues. These abilities make it particularly valuable in the treatment of heart-related injuries and neurodegenerative conditions, where tissue recovery is often limited.

GHK-Cu

- **Collagen Production and Wound Healing**: GHK-Cu, a tripeptide that binds copper, plays a pivotal role in skin health and overall tissue resilience. Because it stimulates collagen synthesis, it restores skin elasticity and reduces visible signs of aging, such as wrinkles and sagging. This peptide also accelerates wound healing, which ensures faster closure of injuries and better-quality tissue regeneration.

- **Skin Regeneration and Anti-Aging**: GHK-Cu supports the repair of skin damage caused by environmental factors and aging, which contributes to smoother, more youthful skin. Its regenerative properties extend beyond cosmetic benefits. It promotes the functional health of skin cells.

Studies on Life Span Extension in Animal Models

Research conducted on animal models has provided invaluable insights into the role of peptides in longevity and overall health. These studies highlight the molecular mechanisms by which specific peptides can positively impact life span and health span. Key findings include:

- **Epitalon and Telomerase Activation**: Research on rodents has suggested that Epitalon may influence telomerase activity, which is an enzyme critical for chromosomal stability, but further studies are needed to confirm its effects on life span extension. This potential activation has been hypothesized to influence cellular aging and immune function, but conclusive evidence on delaying age-related diseases such as cancer is still lacking. The ability of Epitalon to influence these essential biological processes underscores its potential as a tool to address molecular aging.

- **BPC-157**: Animal studies have shown that BPC-157 is highly effective in the promotion of healing of various types of injuries. This includes damage to musculoskeletal tissues as well as gastrointestinal ulcers. Because it accelerates recovery and supports tissue repair, BPC-157 has demonstrated potential to improve long-term health outcomes and mitigate age-related deterioration in these systems.
- **GHK-Cu's Genetic Modulation**: Preliminary research suggests that the peptide GHK-Cu may influence gene expression related to tissue repair and anti-inflammatory responses. It upregulates genes associated with tissue repair and anti-inflammatory responses, which facilitates the body's ability to recover and maintain optimal function. Simultaneously, GHK-Cu downregulates genes linked to oxidative stress, a key contributor to aging and cellular damage. These findings suggest that GHK-Cu may support cellular repair mechanisms, but more research is required to determine its role in combating the effects of aging.

Integrate Peptides into Anti-Aging Protocols

To effectively integrate peptides into anti-aging protocols, a comprehensive and strategic approach is required to maximize benefits and minimize risks. Each aspect of implementation ensures the therapy aligns with the individual's unique needs and promotes optimal outcomes.

Personalization

Anti-aging protocols must be customized to suit individual physiological and biochemical profiles. Biomarkers such as telomere length, levels of inflammatory markers, and mitochondrial function provide critical insights into the aging process for each person.

For Chronic Inflammation: Individuals with elevated inflammatory markers, indicative of persistent inflammation, may benefit most from thymosin beta-4 (TB4). Its ability to regulate immune responses and reduce inflammation can alleviate the effects of inflammaging and prevent further tissue damage.

For Telomere Attrition: Patients who show signs of shortened telomeres, a hallmark of cellular aging, may be considered for Epitalon therapy. While some studies suggest Epitalon may influence telomerase activity, more research is needed to confirm its role in telomere extension and age-related decline.

Administration Methods

The method of peptide administration depends on the peptide's biochemical properties, stability, and the target tissues.

- **Injections**: Many peptides, such as BPC-157 and TB4, are commonly administered via subcutaneous or intramuscular injections to ensure efficient delivery and rapid systemic absorption.

- **Oral Supplementation**: Although less common due to peptide instability in the digestive tract, some formulations have been developed to enhance oral bioavailability for peptides that target broader systemic effects.

- **Topical Applications**: For peptides like GHK-Cu, which promote skin regeneration, topical application ensures direct action on the skin, which makes it effective for localized anti-aging interventions.

Lifestyle Integration

Peptides work most effectively when combined with supportive lifestyle modifications.

- **Exercise**: Regular physical activity enhances peptide therapy because it improves circulation, cellular oxygenation, and overall mitochondrial function, which amplifies the regenerative benefits of peptides.
- **Caloric Restriction**: Controlled caloric intake can reduce oxidative stress and inflammation, which creates a favorable environment for peptides to exert their effects.
- **Nutritional Support**: Nutrients like NAD+ precursors and CoQ10 play a complementary role because they boost energy production and reduce cellular damage, which enhances the effectiveness of peptide therapy.

Safety and Monitoring

Safety and efficacy are paramount when peptide-based anti-aging protocols are implemented.

- **Monitor Continuously:** Regular evaluations, including bloodwork, imaging, and functional tests, are critical to assess the therapy's progress and detect potential side effects early.
- **Individual Response:** It is important to monitor how a patient responds to a specific peptide. This ensures that the therapy remains safe and effective, which allows adjustments to dosages or protocols if necessary. This proactive approach minimizes risks and optimizes long-term outcomes.

Chapter 4: Peptides for Brain Function

Peptides, short chains of amino acids, are essential signaling molecules that regulate numerous biological processes, including brain function. Their role in neuroprotection, cognitive performance enhancement, and the management of neurodegenerative diseases has become a significant focus of research.

Neuroprotective Effects of Peptides

The brain is particularly susceptible to damage from oxidative stress, inflammation, and toxic aggregates, which makes neuroprotection a vital area of focus in neuroscience. Peptides exhibit several mechanisms that protect neurons and maintain brain health.

Combat Oxidative Stress

Oxidative stress occurs when there is an imbalance between the production of ROS and the brain's ability to detoxify these reactive intermediates or repair the damage. This imbalance causes an accumulation of oxidative damage in cellular structures, including lipids, proteins, and DNA. The brain is particularly vulnerable to oxidative stress due to its high oxygen consumption (20% of total body oxygen), abundant lipid content, and relatively low antioxidant defenses.

GSH (glutathione), a tripeptide, is a key component of the brain's antioxidant defenses. While it has an important role in neutralizing ROS and supporting mitochondrial function, it is not classified as a peptide in the same way as signaling peptides that are used in therapeutic applications. Research highlights its depletion as a common feature in neurodegenerative diseases such as Alzheimer's disease (AD) and Parkinson's disease (PD). The administration of GSH precursors like N-acetylcysteine (NAC) has shown promise in the restoration of redox balance.

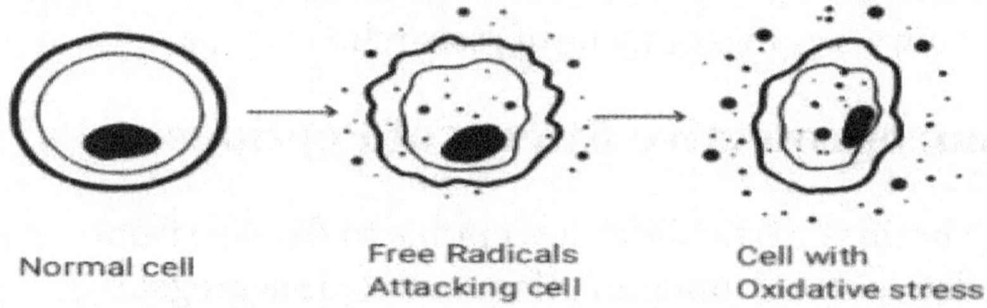

Fig 9: Combat oxidative stress

Anti-Inflammatory Effects

Neuroinflammation refers to the inflammatory response within the central nervous system (CNS), which mainly involves the microglia, astrocytes, endothelial cells, and peripheral immune cells. Although acute neuroinflammation is a protective mechanism aimed at injury or infection, chronic or dysregulated neuroinflammation can lead to neuronal damage, neurodegeneration, and disruption of CNS homeostasis. Chronic neuroinflammation is a hallmark of conditions like AD and amyotrophic lateral sclerosis (ALS).

Peptides such as vasoactive intestinal peptide (VIP) and thymic peptides suppress microglial activation, which reduces the release of pro-inflammatory cytokines. This modulation of the inflammatory response protects neuronal integrity and promotes a healthier brain environment.

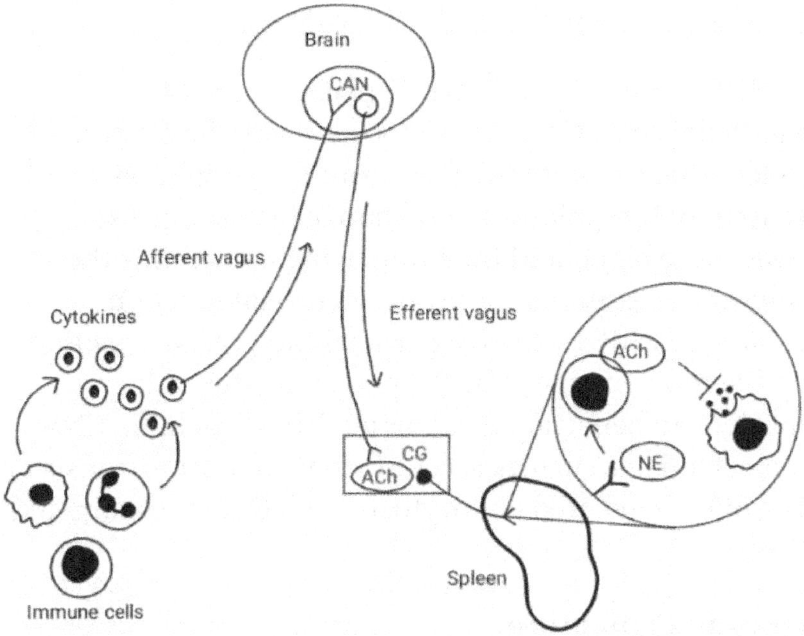

Fig 10: Anti-inflammatory effects

Amyloid-β Plaque Reduction

Amyloid-β (Aβ) plaques are extracellular deposits of aggregated amyloid-β peptides in the brain. They are hallmark pathological features of AD and are implicated in neurodegeneration. The accumulation of these plaques disrupts neuronal communication, triggers neuroinflammation, and contributes to synaptic and neuronal loss. In AD models, VIP has demonstrated neuroprotective effects, but its direct ability to inhibit the formation of amyloid plaques remains under investigation. Through its interaction with amyloid precursors, VIP prevents their aggregation, reduces neuronal death, and preserves cognitive function.

Blood-Brain Barrier (BBB) Crossing

The BBB is a specialized structure composed of endothelial cells, tight junctions, pericytes, and astrocytic end feet that separate the CNS from the peripheral circulation. It regulates the exchange of substances between the blood and the brain, which maintains the homeostasis essential for proper neuronal function. Despite the BBB's selective permeability, certain peptides like diketopiperazines (DKPs) and synthetic cyclic peptides can penetrate this barrier. They reach the CNS via mechanisms such as receptor-mediated transcytosis or adsorption-mediated endocytosis, which ensures targeted delivery.

Synaptic Protection

Synaptic protection refers to the processes and mechanisms that preserve the structure and function of synapses. Synaptic protection is critical for neural circuit integrity, cognitive function, memory, and overall brain health. Neuropeptides enhance synaptic resilience against degenerative processes. For instance, studies have shown that GLP-1 analogs and other peptides promote synapse preservation in preclinical models of neurodegenerative diseases.

Peptides Enhance Cognitive Performance

Cognitive enhancement refers to the process of improved mental functions such as memory, attention, executive function, creativity, and decision-making through various methods, including pharmacological, behavioral, or technological interventions. These enhancements are used in both clinical and nonclinical settings to optimize brain function.

Cognitive enhancement through peptides involves mechanisms that boost memory, learning, and attention. These effects stem from their ability to influence neurotransmitter systems, neuronal plasticity, and overall brain health.

Neurotransmitter Regulation

Neurotransmitters are chemical messengers that transmit signals across synapses between neurons. Proper regulation of neurotransmitter levels, release, and receptor activity is fundamental to cognitive processes like memory, attention, learning, and executive function. Dysregulation of neurotransmitters is linked to cognitive deficits, while targeted modulation can enhance cognitive performance. Peptides play a vital role in the modulation of neurotransmitters like dopamine, acetylcholine, and glutamate, which are critical for cognitive processes. For example, GLP-1 analogs not only improve insulin sensitivity in neurons but also stimulate dopamine release, which enhances motivation and attention.

Peptides that Boost Memory

Dietary-derived peptides, such as those found in fermented dairy products, improve cognitive functions because they influence synaptic signaling pathways. Animal studies have demonstrated significant improvements in learning and memory with the administration of these peptides.

Enhance Synaptic Plasticity

Peptides like brain-derived neurotrophic factor (BDNF) mimic natural neurotrophic factors that enhance synaptic strength and promote long-term potentiation, a process essential for learning and memory. Studies on apamin, a venom-derived peptide, have revealed its neuroprotective effects on synaptic transmission in damaged neurons. Similarly, cyclic peptides derived from milk proteins show high permeability across the BBB and have demonstrated cognitive benefits in animal models. Some examples of neuroactive peptides that are investigated for their potential cognitive benefits are listed below.

Semax

Derived from an adrenocorticotropic hormone (ACTH) fragment, Semax enhances cognitive functions such as attention, learning, and memory. It increases BDNF expression, which is essential for neuronal health. Semax is clinically used in some countries for cognitive enhancement purposes.

Cerebrolysin

A peptide mixture derived from brain proteins that supports neurogenesis and neuronal survival, it has clinical applications in stroke recovery and has shown evidence of improved cognitive function in elderly populations.

Role of Peptides in Neurodegenerative Disease Management

Neurodegenerative diseases are a group of disorders characterized by the progressive degeneration or death of neurons in the central or peripheral nervous system. They often lead to cognitive, motor, and behavioral impairments, based on the regions of the nervous system affected. Examples include AD, PD, Huntington's disease (HD), and ALS.

Peptides play a significant role in the pathogenesis of neurodegenerative diseases, often through mechanisms involving protein aggregation, toxicity, and disruption of normal cellular functions. The accumulation and misfolding of specific peptides are central to disease progression.

Alzheimer's Disease

AD is a neurological illness that mainly affects older persons and is characterized by behavioral abnormalities, memory loss, and cognitive impairment. The pathogenesis of AD is heavily influenced by the accumulation of two key peptides: amyloid beta (Aβ) and tau protein. Amyloid beta, especially the Aβ42 form, is cleaved from the amyloid precursor protein and aggregates to form amyloid plaques in the brain's extracellular space. These plaques disrupt neuronal function, trigger inflammation, and lead to oxidative stress, which contributes to neuronal damage and cognitive decline. Meanwhile, tau, a protein that normally stabilizes microtubules, becomes hyperphosphorylated in AD and forms twisted tangles inside neurons. These neurofibrillary tangles impair intracellular transport and further contribute to neuronal dysfunction and death. The combined effects of amyloid plaques and tau tangles result in progressive damage to the brain's structures, particularly in areas responsible for memory, which causes the hallmark symptoms of AD.

However, there is some evidence that certain peptides, particularly in their earlier or non-aggregated forms, may play protective roles in the brain. VIP and GLP-1 analogs reduce amyloid-β accumulation and tau hyperphosphorylation, both key pathological markers of AD. Because they inhibit these processes, peptides protect synapses and enhance cognitive function.

Clinical Potential: Preclinical studies suggest that VIP may have neuroprotective effects, but its direct ability to reduce hippocampal and cortical atrophy in humans remains under investigation.

Parkinson's Disease

PD is a progressive neurodegenerative disorder mainly characterized by motor symptoms such as tremors, rigidity, bradykinesia, and postural instability, often accompanied by non-motor symptoms like cognitive decline and mood disorders. The pathogenesis of PD is mainly linked to the degeneration of dopaminergic neurons in the substantia nigra, a region of the brain involved in movement control. The aggregation of α-synuclein, a protein that creates toxic clumps called Lewy bodies inside neurons, is a major factor in the development of the disease. Because dopamine is necessary to regulate movement, these aggregates impair normal cell function and cause neuronal death, with an eventual decrease in dopamine synthesis. Although α-synuclein aggregation is generally detrimental, there is evidence that small amounts of α-synuclein in its native, non-aggregated form may play a protective role because they regulate synaptic vesicle trafficking and dopamine release.

Additionally, certain peptides involved in the regulation of oxidative stress and inflammation, such as BDNF, may provide neuroprotection in the early stages of the disease because they promote neuronal survival and repair mechanisms. However, when these peptides are dysregulated or overwhelmed by the toxic effects of α-synuclein aggregates, they lose their protective capabilities, which contributes to the progression of Parkinson's disease.

GLP-1 receptor agonists have shown potential neuroprotective effects on dopaminergic neurons, reducing oxidative stress and apoptosis, but VIP's role in Parkinson's disease remains less clearly defined. GLP-1 receptor agonists have also been shown to improve motor function in preclinical models. Peptides that target insulin resistance in the brain, such as GLP-1 receptor agonists, have shown potential for improving neuronal survival and motor function, but their direct effect on dopamine synthesis remains under study.

Amyotrophic Lateral Sclerosis (ALS)

ALS affects motor neurons and results in muscle weakening, paralysis, and eventual respiratory failure. ALS is characterized by the degeneration of both upper motor neurons (in the brain) and lower motor neurons (in the spinal cord), which control voluntary muscles. The pathogenesis of ALS is linked to various factors, including the accumulation of abnormal proteins such as superoxide dismutase 1 (SOD1), TAR DNA-binding protein 43 (TDP-43), and fused-in sarcoma (FUS). SOD1 mutations, for instance, lead to misfolded SOD1 proteins that aggregate within motor neurons. This disrupts cellular processes and promotes oxidative stress, mitochondrial dysfunction, and inflammation. TDP-43, another key protein, usually binds RNA but becomes mislocalized and forms toxic aggregates in ALS, which disrupts RNA processing and protein homeostasis. In ALS, these protein aggregates are thought to play a critical role in motor neuron degeneration, which contributes to the loss of muscle control.

Peptides like VIP mitigate motor neuron degeneration because they suppress neuroinflammatory processes. Certain peptides, such as GLP-1 receptor agonists, have shown promise in ALS models for improving motor function and neuroprotection, but their effect on overall survival is still under investigation.

Huntington's Disease

HD is a hereditary neurodegenerative disorder caused by a mutation in the huntingtin gene, which causes the production of an abnormal form of the huntingtin protein. This mutant protein contains an expanded polyglutamine (polyQ) tract, which causes the protein to misfold and aggregate. This forms intranuclear inclusions in neurons. The pathogenesis of HD is linked to these toxic aggregates of huntingtin, which disrupt normal cellular functions because they interfere with transcription, protein degradation, and mitochondrial function. The accumulation of huntingtin aggregates mainly affects the basal ganglia, a brain region responsible for movement control, which causes motor symptoms such as chorea (involuntary jerky movements), dystonia, and eventual progressive motor and cognitive decline. These toxic aggregates also lead to neuronal death and a gradual loss of cognitive and motor function, which is characteristic of HD. Although mutant huntingtin is toxic, there is ongoing research into potential therapeutic strategies aimed at the reduction of its aggregation or the degradation of misfolded proteins to slow the progression of the disease. In HD, antisense oligonucleotide-based therapies target mutant huntingtin mRNA, which reduces the production of toxic huntingtin protein aggregates in neurons.

Multiple Sclerosis (MS)

Multiple sclerosis (MS) is a chronic autoimmune disease of the CNS characterized by the immune system's attacks on the myelin sheath, a protective cover around nerve fibers. This results in inflammation, demyelination, and subsequent axonal damage, which causes a range of neurological symptoms such as fatigue, muscle weakness, numbness, vision problems, and cognitive dysfunction. The pathogenesis of MS is complex and involves both genetic and environmental factors. The immune system mistakenly targets myelin as if it were a foreign invader. Key peptides implicated in the disease include myelin basic protein, proteolipid protein, and myelin oligodendrocyte glycoprotein, which are components of the myelin sheath. In MS, these peptides become the target of autoantibodies and activated T cells, which attack and damage the myelin, which causes inflammation and plaques in the CNS. The resultant demyelination slows or blocks nerve signal transmission, which causes the neurological symptoms associated with MS. Although the immune response is harmful in MS, there is some evidence that peptides like T regulatory cell-derived cytokines may play a protective role because they regulate the immune response and limit the extent of autoimmune damage. However, in MS, the immune system's dysregulation outweighs these protective mechanisms, which causes ongoing damage to the myelin and neurons. GLP-1 receptor agonists have shown potential neuroprotective effects in preclinical MS models, but their direct role for reducing CNS inflammation and demyelination requires further clinical validation. They also improve vascular health, which mitigates secondary complications.

Mechanism of Peptides in Synaptic Plasticity and Memory

Synaptic plasticity underpins learning and memory, and peptides influence this process in several ways.

- **TrkB Pathway Activation:** BDNF-mimetic peptides activate the TrkB receptor, which enhances synaptic strength and promotes long-term potentiation. This pathway is central to memory formation and retention.

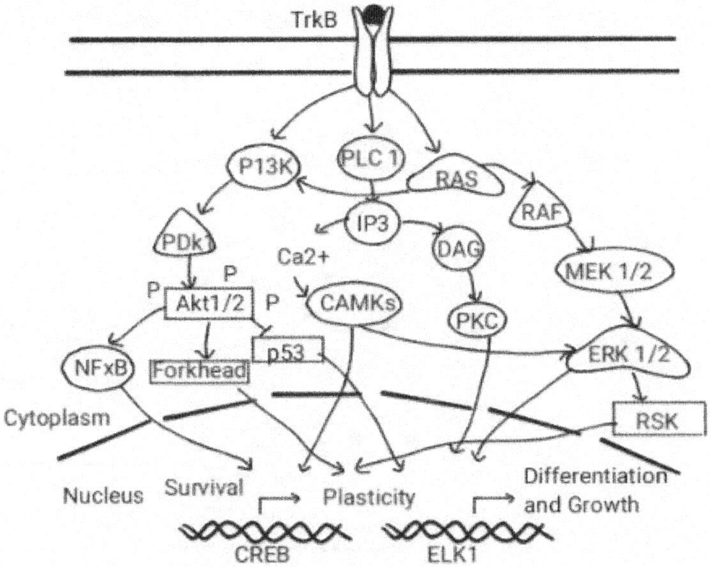

Fig 11: TrkB pathway activation

- **Calcium Ion Regulation:** Peptides modulate calcium channels, which are essential for neurotransmitter release and synaptic signaling. Dysregulation of calcium homeostasis is a common feature in neurodegenerative diseases.

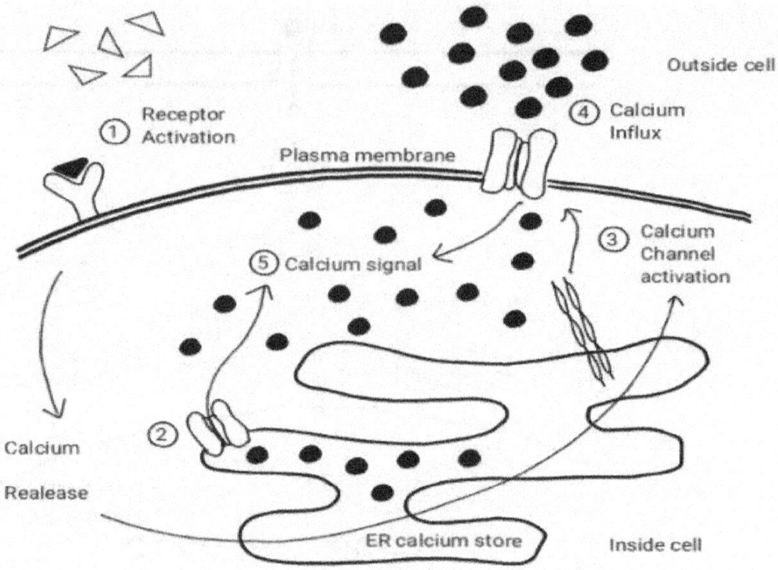

Fig 12: Calcium ion regulation

- **Structural Synaptic Changes:** Because they promote dendritic spine growth and stability, peptides like BDNF and GLP-1 receptor agonists support synaptic connections, which enhances neural networks responsible for cognition.
- **Interaction with α-amino-3-hydroxy-5-methyl-4-isoxazolepropionic Acid Receptors (AMPA) and N-methyl-D-aspartate (NMDA) Receptors:** Peptides enhance the activity of glutamate receptors, which is critical for excitatory synaptic transmission and memory encoding.

Peptides Modulate Mood and Mental Health

Peptides play a critical role in the modulation of mood and mental health because they influence various biochemical pathways and signaling mechanisms in the brain. Several key peptides have been identified as essential players in emotional regulation, stress response, and overall mental well-being.

One of the most well-known peptides involved in mood regulation is oxytocin, often referred to as the love hormone. Oxytocin is heavily implicated in social bonding, trust, and emotional regulation. It has been shown to reduce stress, promote positive social interactions, and improve mood in both humans and animals. Oxytocin's effects on bonding and attachment are particularly important in relationships and emotional well-being, and its release is associated with feelings of comfort and connection.

Another important group of peptides is the endorphins, which act as natural painkillers and mood enhancers. Endorphins are released during physical activity, laughter, social bonding, and even in response to pain. They play a vital role in stress reduction, alleviate pain, and promote feelings of pleasure and happiness. As endogenous opioids, endorphins help regulate mood because they enhance positive emotions and minimize feelings of discomfort.

On the flip side, corticotropin-releasing hormone (CRH) is a peptide involved in the body's response to stress. Elevated levels of CRH are associated with anxiety, depression, and other mood disorders. CRH promotes a heightened stress response because it stimulates the release of cortisol, the body's primary stress hormone. Dysregulation of CRH levels can contribute to chronic stress and exacerbate mood disorders.

Neuropeptide Y (NPY) is another peptide that has a protective effect on mental health. NPY regulates stress, anxiety, and emotional resilience. Higher levels of NPY are linked to reduced anxiety and improved resilience to stress. Research suggests that NPY may also help counteract the effects of disorders like depression and post-traumatic stress disorder because it stabilizes the nervous system's response to stress.

Vasopressin and somatostatin are additional peptides that influence mood and mental health. Vasopressin plays a role in social behaviors and stress responses, influencing emotional regulation, social bonding, and aggression, with both prosocial and stress-amplifying effects depending on context and receptor activation. Elevated vasopressin levels are often found in individuals with social anxiety and depression. On the other hand, somatostatin exerts inhibitory effects on neurotransmitter release, particularly on growth hormone and corticotropin-releasing hormone (CRH), which can influence mood, stress response, and cognition. It has been suggested that alterations in somatostatin functioning may contribute to mood disorders because they disrupt neurotransmitter balance in the brain. Peptides influence mood and mental health through their actions on stress, anxiety, depression, and sleep regulation.

Ethical Considerations and Potential Abuse

As peptide therapies advance, ethical concerns and the potential for misuse must be addressed.

- **Regulatory Oversight:** The unregulated sale of synthetic peptides raises concerns about quality, safety, and efficacy.
- **Performance Enhancement Misuse:** Peptides marketed for cognitive or athletic enhancement may be abused, particularly in competitive environments.
- **Access and Equity:** The high cost of peptide therapies could exacerbate health disparities and limit access to vulnerable populations.
- **Long-Term Safety:** Although peptides provide targeted benefits, their long-term effects on brain function and systemic health remain underexplored.

Chapter 5: Peptides for Immunity

Peptides play a critical role in immune modulation and provide applications in antiviral defense, autoimmune disease treatment, and vaccine development. Their ability to interact with immune cell receptors and signaling pathways makes them valuable tools in immunotherapy.

Role of Peptides in Immune Modulation

Peptides influence immune responses through direct interaction with immune cells and modulate cytokine production. They enhance macrophage activity, stimulate T and B lymphocytes, and regulate inflammatory response.

Interaction with Immune Cells

Certain peptides, such as lactoferrin-derived peptides, modulate immune cell activity because they bind to specific receptors on neutrophils, macrophages, and natural killer (NK) cells. These interactions result in increased phagocytosis, cytokine production, and overall immune system activation. Lactoferrin-derived peptides enhance the ability of macrophages to engulf and destroy pathogens through the upregulation of key signaling pathways, such as the NF-κB and MAPK pathways, which causes the production of pro-inflammatory cytokines like TNF-α and IL-6. Additionally, these peptides promote the secretion of chemokines that attract other immune cells to the site of infection, further amplifying the immune response. NK cells, which play a critical role in antiviral and anticancer immunity, also exhibit increased cytotoxic activity in response to lactoferrin-derived peptides, which causes the enhanced destruction of infected or malignant cells. Because they stimulate these immune mechanisms, lactoferrin-derived peptides contribute significantly to the body's ability to defend against a wide range of pathogens.

Cytokine Modulation

Peptides can regulate cytokine expression, which influences both inflammatory and anti-inflammatory responses. For example, lactoferrin-derived peptides play a dual role. They balance pro-inflammatory and anti-inflammatory cytokines, which is critical for immune homeostasis. These peptides inhibit the overproduction of pro-inflammatory cytokines such as TNF-α and IL-6, which are commonly associated with excessive immune responses that cause chronic inflammation and autoimmune diseases. This inhibition occurs through the modulation of intracellular signaling pathways such as NF-κB and JAK-STAT, which are critical in cytokine gene expression.

Simultaneously, lactoferrin-derived peptides enhance the secretion of anti-inflammatory cytokines like IL-10, which helps suppress excessive immune responses and promote tissue repair. IL-10 downregulates antigen-presenting cell activity and limits the production of pro-inflammatory mediators. This prevents tissue damage and autoimmunity. Additionally, these peptides can influence T-regulatory cells (Tregs), which play a significant role in immune tolerance and the resolution of inflammation. Because they stimulate IL-10 production and Treg activity, lactoferrin-derived peptides contribute to an overall immunomodulatory effect, which makes them valuable candidates for therapeutic interventions in inflammatory and autoimmune conditions.

Peptides Enhance Antiviral and Antimicrobial Defense

Antimicrobial peptides (AMPs) serve as the body's first line of defense against pathogens because they exhibit broad-spectrum antibacterial, antiviral, and antifungal properties. These peptides play a critical role in innate immunity because they disrupt microbial membranes, neutralize toxins, and modulate immune cell responses.

Nursing Implications

- Closely monitor patients who receive peptide-based immunotherapies for signs of altered immune responses, such as excessive inflammation or inadequate immune activation. Watch for changes in vital signs, fever, or local reactions at the injection site.

- Understand that peptides modulate both pro-inflammatory and anti-inflammatory cytokines, so nurses must be vigilant for symptoms of cytokine imbalance, which could lead to complications such as chronic inflammation or immunosuppression.

- Educate patients about how these peptides work. Inform them about potential side effects and why they should report any unexpected symptoms promptly.

- Work closely with the healthcare team to ensure they regularly monitor laboratory markers (e.g., inflammatory markers) and adjust care plans as needed. This ensures that the immunomodulatory therapy achieves its intended benefits with minimal adverse effects.

Mechanism of Action

AMPs function through various mechanisms, including direct microbial membrane disruption, inhibition of intracellular processes, and modulation of host immune responses. Many AMPs, such as LL-37, achieve bacterial lysis because they integrate into microbial membranes and form pores that lead to cell death. LL-37 also interferes with viral replication because it binds to viral envelopes and prevents their entry into host cells, which makes it an effective defense mechanism against viral infections.

Examples of Antimicrobial Peptides

- **Lactoferrin-derived peptides**: These peptides enhance phagocytosis, neutralize bacterial toxins, and exhibit potent antimicrobial properties because they chelate iron, which is essential for bacterial growth. They also disrupt bacterial membranes and inhibit pathogen adhesion to host cells, reducing infection risk.

- **Defensins**: Found in epithelial cells and neutrophils, defensins protect against bacterial and viral infections because they disrupt pathogen membranes and activate immune cells. They also play a role in cytokine production, which supports an effective immune response.

- **Cathelicidins (e.g., LL-37)**: These peptides act as potent antimicrobial agents that destroy bacterial membranes, inhibit biofilm formation, and neutralize endotoxins. LL-37 is particularly significant due to its dual role in the direct elimination of pathogens. It also modulates immune responses because it enhances chemotaxis and cytokine production.

Applications in Autoimmune Disease Treatment

Peptides provide novel therapeutic approaches for autoimmune diseases because they modulate immune responses and induce tolerance.

Peptide-Based Immunotherapy

Peptide-based therapies aim to restore immune balance because they target autoreactive T cells. For example, synthetic peptide analogs mimic self-antigens to induce immune tolerance, which reduces autoimmune attacks. These therapies selectively modulate T-cell responses, suppress autoreactive lymphocytes, and preserve overall immune function. These precision peptide-based therapies have become a focus in autoimmune disease treatment, as they can modulate immune responses in a targeted manner. In MS, peptides that mimic myelin epitopes help reduce autoreactive T-cell activity, which prevents demyelination and preserves nerve function.

This is critical to limit nerve damage and functional decline.

For rheumatoid arthritis, peptide-based treatments suppress the inflammatory response. They modulate T-cell activation, which reduces joint inflammation and slows disease progression. Because they specifically target immune cells that drive inflammation, these therapies may provide more tailored and effective relief.

In type 1 diabetes, immunomodulatory peptides help balance immune responses against pancreatic beta cells. They have the potential to reduce disease severity and delay the onset of insulin dependence because they prevent destructive immune activity.

These approaches are designed to target specific pathways responsible for disease progression. This provides a way to treat the root cause rather than just the symptoms and could revolutionize the management of autoimmune diseases in the future.

In MS, peptides mimic myelin epitopes to interact with autoreactive T-cells, which mistakenly attack the myelin around nerve fibers. Because they modulate these T-cells, peptide-based treatments help prevent demyelination, protect nerve function, and slow disease progression.

Peptide-based therapies provide a targeted approach to treat various autoimmune diseases through the modulation of the immune system with greater precision. In MS, for instance, peptides designed to mimic specific myelin epitopes interact with autoreactive T-cells that erroneously attack the myelin sheath surrounding nerve fibers. Because they induce immune tolerance or modify T-cell activation, these peptides help prevent demyelination, preserve nerve function, and ultimately slow disease progression.

Similarly, in rheumatoid arthritis, peptide-based treatments dampen the inflammatory responses that lead to joint damage. These peptides modulate T-cell activation, a critical driver of inflammation in the joints. As a result, they reduce the severity of joint inflammation, alleviate pain, and help slow down the degradation of cartilage and bone, which provides a more focused treatment strategy compared to conventional immunosuppressants.

In type 1 diabetes, immunomodulatory peptides aim to control the autoimmune response against pancreatic beta cells. Because they regulate T-cell activity, these peptides reduce the intensity of the immune attack on beta cells, which preserves their function. This can help reduce disease severity and potentially delay the onset of the condition.

Peptide-based therapies represent an innovative approach and provide disease-specific interventions that may provide improved outcomes and reduced side effects compared to traditional therapies. They help minimize side effects compared to conventional immunosuppressive treatments.

Mechanisms of Action on Immune Cell Signaling Pathways

Peptides influence immune responses through key signaling pathways that regulate cell activation, proliferation, and cytokine secretion. These pathways include:

- **Toll-Like Receptor (TLR) Signaling:** TLRs are essential components of the innate immune system. They recognize pathogen-associated molecular patterns. Some peptides can directly interact with TLRs or influence their downstream signaling, which enhances the immune system's ability to detect and respond to invading pathogens. Because they modulate TLR pathways, peptides not only amplify the production of pro-inflammatory cytokines required for effective pathogen clearance but also help maintain self-tolerance, which prevents excessive or autoimmune responses.

- **Major Histocompatibility Complex (MHC) Presentation:**
  Peptides are central to antigen processing and presentation. When bound to MHC molecules on the surface of antigen-presenting cells, these peptides are recognized by T cells, which determines whether an immune response is activated or suppressed. This selective presentation is vital to ensure that the immune system targets pathogenic antigens and avoids self-antigens. This refines the specificity and balance of T-cell

responses. Certain peptides can be engineered to enhance this process, which makes them good candidates in immunotherapy.

- **JAK-STAT Signaling:** Many cytokines signal through the JAK-STAT pathway, a critical conduit to translate extracellular signals into gene expression changes that drive immune responses. Peptides that mimic cytokines or act as inhibitors can regulate this pathway. They modulate the balance between pro-inflammatory and anti-inflammatory signals. This control is essential for immune homeostasis and ensures a measured response during infection or inflammation.
- **NF-κB and MAPK Pathways:** Both NF-κB and MAPK pathways are central regulators of immune cell survival, proliferation, and the production of inflammatory mediators. Peptides can either activate these pathways, which causes an upregulation of cytokine production and immune cell proliferation, or suppress them, which reduces inflammation. This dual functionality allows peptides to tailor immune responses to the specific context, which promotes effective pathogen clearance and minimizes tissue damage.

Challenges in Peptide-Based Immunotherapy

Despite their potential, peptide-based immunotherapies face several challenges, including stability, delivery, and immune tolerance.

Stability and Degradation

Peptides are prone to enzymatic degradation, which reduces their efficacy before they reach their intended targets. Strategies to enhance stability include chemical modifications such as cyclization, PEGylation, and incorporation of non-natural amino acids, which improve peptide half-life and bioavailability. Additionally, structural modifications like peptide stapling and backbone cyclization help preserve biological activity and prevent rapid enzymatic breakdown.

Delivery Challenges

Efficient delivery systems are essential for peptide-based therapies to be effective. Nanoparticles and liposomes are increasingly being explored as carriers to enhance peptide bioavailability, target specificity, and sustained release. These delivery platforms protect peptides from enzymatic degradation and ensure their controlled release at the site of action. Other approaches include hydrogels, microneedles, and implantable peptide-release systems, which facilitate localized and prolonged therapeutic effects.

Immune Tolerance and Immunogenicity

Repeated exposure to therapeutic peptides can sometimes induce immune tolerance rather than activation, which reduces their effectiveness. To address this, researchers have designed peptides with optimized antigenic properties. They've incorporated adjuvants and used novel delivery mechanisms to enhance immune activation and minimize undesired immune suppression. Personalized peptide vaccines, which tailor peptide sequences to an individual's immune profile, are also being explored to maximize therapeutic efficacy and avoid unwanted tolerance.

Research Trends in Immunopeptides

Recent research focuses on peptide-based therapies enhanced through computational design, novel delivery methods, and synthetic biology.

Computational Peptide Design

Computational models and artificial intelligence are utilized to predict peptide structures, optimize binding affinities, and design more stable immunogenic peptides. Machine-learning algorithms help analyze vast datasets of peptide interactions with immune receptors, which accelerates the discovery of highly specific and effective therapeutic peptides.

Novel Delivery Methods

Advancements in peptide delivery technologies aim to improve stability, bioavailability, and targeting efficiency. Nanoparticle-based delivery systems, including lipid nanoparticles and polymeric nanoparticles, protect peptides from enzymatic degradation and ensure controlled release. Additionally, microneedle patches and hydrogel-based delivery systems provide minimally invasive administration methods that enhance peptide absorption and efficacy.

Synthetic Biology Approaches

Synthetic biology has revolutionized peptide-based immunotherapy because it enables the design of synthetic peptides with enhanced immunogenicity and specificity. Engineered peptides with modified amino acid sequences exhibit improved resistance to proteolysis, which ensures longer circulation times and sustained therapeutic effects. Furthermore, synthetic biology approaches facilitate the development of multi-epitope peptide vaccines that target multiple immune pathways simultaneously, which increases overall efficacy.

Peptide-Based Nanoparticle Vaccines

Self-assembling peptide nanoparticles improve antigen stability and immune response, which advances peptide-based vaccine strategies. These nanoparticles mimic viral structures, enhance antigen presentation, and promote robust immune activation. Because they improve peptide stability and prolong circulation time, nanoparticle-based vaccines ensure a sustained immune response. Furthermore, peptide nanoparticles allow for targeted delivery, which reduces potential side effects and maximizes efficacy. Researchers have begun to explore multi-epitope peptide nanoparticle vaccines that combine multiple antigens to provide broader protection against infections and diseases. These advances in peptide-based nanotechnology hold great promise for next-generation vaccines and immunotherapies.

Nursing Implications

Peptides that modulate immune cell signaling pathways, such as those that affect TLR signaling, MHC presentation, the JAK-STAT cascade, and the NF-κB and MAPK pathways, are important agents in both diagnostic and therapeutic settings. For nurses, knowledge of the mechanisms by which these peptides act is essential to safely administer these therapies, monitor patient responses, and educate patients about what to expect during treatment.

Administer and Monitor

Dose and Route of Administration

Peptide therapies are often administered via injection or infusion, and their dose may be adjusted based on the desired immunomodulatory effect. Nurses must ensure that the correct dose is administered via the appropriate route, following established protocols. They must also be familiar with any pre-administration guidelines that accompany these agents, such as premedication to prevent allergic reactions.

Monitor for Adverse Reactions

Due to their potent effects on the immune system, peptide immunotherapies can cause a range of adverse reactions. Nursing responsibilities include:

- **Observation for Allergic Reactions:** Monitor for signs of hypersensitivity, such as swelling, hives, or difficulty breathing.

- **Infusion-Related Reactions:** Watch for changes in blood pressure, heart rate, or temperature during and after the administration of peptides.
- **Laboratory Monitoring:** Regularly review complete blood counts, inflammatory markers (e.g., C-reactive protein), and specific cytokine levels, if indicated, to assess the patient's response to therapy.
- **Documentation:** Accurately and thoroughly document all patient responses and any adverse events. This is critical for the evaluation and adjustment of therapy.

Patient Education and Communication

Explain the Therapy

Patients who receive peptide immunotherapies should be informed about how these agents work. Nurses can explain that the peptides are designed to adjust immune system signals and either enhance the ability to fight infections or temper an overactive immune response in conditions such as autoimmune disorders. This education helps patients understand both the benefits and the potential side effects.

Set Expectations

Patients should be counseled on what to expect after they receive the peptides. This includes possible side effects, such as injection site reactions, transient flu-like symptoms, or mild fever. Patients need to know when these symptoms are expected and when to seek medical advice.

Self-Monitor and Report

Nurses should empower patients to monitor their symptoms. For example, patients should be instructed to report any signs of an allergic reaction immediately and to keep a log of any unusual symptoms or changes in their overall well-being. This proactive approach ensures that any adverse effects are managed promptly.

Special Considerations for Different Patient Populations

Immunocompromised Patients

Patients with weakened immune systems may respond differently to peptide therapies. Nurses need to assess baseline immune status and monitor these patients more closely for signs of infection or over-suppression. Therapy adjustments may be necessary to ensure that the benefits outweigh the risks.

Patients with Autoimmune Disorders

For patients with autoimmune conditions, peptides that modulate immune cell signaling can be particularly beneficial. However, these patients may also be more susceptible to adverse effects if the balance between pro-inflammatory and anti-inflammatory signals is disrupted. Nurses must carefully observe patients for any exacerbation of autoimmune symptoms and communicate promptly with the medical team.

Pediatric and Geriatric Populations

Age-related changes in immune function necessitate special dose considerations. In pediatric patients, precise doses and vigilant observation are critical. In geriatric patients, coexisting conditions and polypharmacy require that nurses pay close attention to potential drug interactions and age-related pharmacodynamic changes.

Chapter 6: Peptides for Hormonal Health

Peptides have an outsized impact on human physiology. They serve as messengers and regulators throughout the body, particularly within the endocrine system, where precise hormonal control is essential for homeostasis. Over the past century, peptides have moved from simple replacement therapies to complex, engineered molecules that fine-tune hormonal regulation and treat a wide range of disorders.

Mechanism of Peptides in Hormonal Regulation

At the core of hormonal regulation is the intricate interplay between peptide ligands and their specific cell surface receptors. Peptides act as signaling molecules that bind with high specificity to receptors on target cells. This binding often triggers a cascade of intracellular events, frequently via second messenger systems such as cyclic AMP (cAMP), phospholipase C, or MAPK. This ultimately alters gene expression, enzyme activity, or ion channel function.

A classic example is the interaction between adropin, a peptide involved in metabolic regulation, and its putative receptor(s). Although much remains to be elucidated about adropin's receptor binding, studies have shown that this peptide modulates metabolic processes because it influences adipocyte proliferation and lipid metabolism. The ability of peptides to rapidly modulate cellular function makes them ideal to fine-tune endocrine processes. Unlike larger proteins, peptides generally have shorter half-lives, which ensures that their actions are swift and transient. This rapid turnover is particularly important in systems where a quick adjustment is needed, such as during the regulation of blood glucose or stress responses.

Peptide hormones are synthesized and secreted in a pulsatile manner. For instance, the secretion of hypothalamic-releasing hormones is tightly regulated to stimulate or inhibit downstream hormone production in the pituitary gland. This pulsatility is critical because it ensures that target cells do not become desensitized to constant stimulation. In many cases, the peptide's structure is amenable to chemical modifications, which allows pharmaceutical scientists to engineer analogs with improved stability, longer half-life, or enhanced receptor specificity. Such advancements have paved the way for the development of therapeutic agents that mimic natural peptides and overcome the limitations of rapid degradation in vivo.

Peptides Address Growth Hormone Deficiencies

GH plays a pivotal role in normal growth, metabolism, and tissue repair. Deficiencies in GH, whether congenital or acquired, can lead to growth disorders in children and metabolic disturbances in adults. Therapeutic approaches with peptide analogs focus on two main strategies: stimulating the release of endogenous GH and replacing the deficient hormone itself.

GHRH and its Analogs

GHRH is a hypothalamic peptide that binds to receptors on pituitary somatotrophs to promote the secretion of GH. Synthetic analogs of GHRH, such as sermorelin, have been developed to stimulate GH release in individuals with deficiencies. These peptides mimic the structure and function of natural GHRH, which causes increased pituitary secretion of GH. Because they enhance the body's own GH production, GHRH analogs can promote more physiological growth patterns and metabolic balance compared to direct hormone replacement.

Growth Hormone-Releasing Peptides (GHRPs)

Complementary to GHRH analogs, GHRPs such as GHRP-2, GHRP-6, and Ipamorelin have emerged as another class of agents to combat GH deficiency. GHRPs act on different receptors than GHRH, sometimes in concert with ghrelin receptors, to stimulate GH secretion. Their mechanism of action binds to receptors that, upon activation, increase intracellular calcium levels and trigger exocytosis of GH-containing vesicles. Clinical studies have shown that GHRPs can not only augment GH release but may also improve the pulsatility of GH secretion, which is critical for optimal metabolic effects.

The therapeutic utility of these peptides lies in their ability to restore a more normal endocrine milieu without daily injections of recombinant GH. Moreover, because these peptides stimulate endogenous GH production, they tend to preserve the natural feedback mechanisms that regulate hormone levels. Research across several decades, from early isolation techniques described in historical reviews to modern synthetic methods, has refined these peptides to maximize efficacy and minimize side effects such as insulin resistance or edema.

Nursing Implications

- Regularly assess growth parameters, metabolic indicators, and signs of improved tissue repair in children and adults who receive peptide therapies.
- Monitor for side effects such as insulin resistance or edema.
- Ensure correct dosing and timely administration of GHRH analogs or GHRPs.
- Educate patients and caregivers on proper injection techniques and storage of peptide medications.
- Explain how these peptides stimulate endogenous GH production, which helps to restore natural hormonal balance.
- Inform patients about the importance of adherence to therapy and routine follow-ups to monitor treatment efficacy.
- Work closely with endocrinologists to adjust therapy based on clinical response and laboratory findings.
- Document and communicate any adverse effects or changes in patient condition for timely intervention.

Role of Peptides in Insulin and Glucose Levels

Diabetes and metabolic syndrome are characterized by dysregulated insulin secretion and impaired glucose homeostasis. In recent years, peptide hormones have emerged as critical players in the management of these conditions. The incretin system, particularly GLP-1 and glucose-dependent insulinotropic polypeptide, exemplifies how peptides can influence insulin dynamics and overall energy balance.

Incretin Hormones and Their Mechanisms

Incretins are secreted by the gut in response to food intake. GLP-1, for example, binds to receptors on pancreatic β-cells, which causes an increase in intracellular cAMP. This activation promotes insulin secretion in a glucose-dependent manner, which means that insulin release is amplified only when blood glucose levels are elevated. Such a mechanism not only enhances postprandial insulin secretion but also reduces the risk of hypoglycemia. Additionally, GLP-1 slows gastric emptying and suppresses glucagon secretion, which further contributes to improved glycemic control.

Pharmaceutical developments have capitalized on these properties. Modified analogs of GLP-1, such as exenatide and liraglutide, have been engineered to resist rapid enzymatic degradation, which prolongs their action and allows for less frequent dosing. These drugs have become a cornerstone in the management of type 2 diabetes. They provide benefits that extend beyond glucose control to include weight loss and cardiovascular protection.

Peptides in Insulin Sensitivity and Metabolic Regulation

Beyond incretins, other peptides contribute to insulin sensitivity and overall metabolic balance. For example, peptides like adropin play a role in the modulation of lipid metabolism and insulin sensitivity. Although research on adropin continues, initial findings suggest that higher levels of adropin are associated with improved insulin sensitivity and reduced adiposity. Such insights open avenues for peptide analogs to be used as therapeutic agents in metabolic syndrome, where insulin resistance is a central feature.

Nursing Implications

- Regularly monitor blood glucose levels, weight, and cardiovascular parameters to assess the effectiveness of peptide therapies in the management of type 2 diabetes and metabolic syndrome.
- Watch for any adverse reactions, including signs of hypoglycemia or gastrointestinal discomfort.
- Educate patients on how peptide-based treatments, such as GLP-1 analogs, work to enhance insulin secretion, slow gastric emptying, and improve insulin sensitivity.
- Inform patients about the benefits, such as reduced hypoglycemia risk, potential weight loss, and cardiovascular protection, as well as possible side effects.

- Ensure proper administration techniques, whether injections or other delivery methods, and emphasize adherence to the dosing schedule.
- Instruct patients on the proper storage of peptide medications to maintain efficacy.
- Collaborate with endocrinologists, dietitians, and pharmacists to optimize treatment plans based on individual patient needs and monitor overall metabolic status.
- Accurately document patient responses, lab values, and any side effects to facilitate timely adjustments in therapy.
- Schedule regular follow-ups to evaluate treatment outcomes and reinforce patient education on self-monitoring practices.

Thyrotropin-Releasing Hormone (TRH) and Thyroid Regulation

TRH is synthesized in the hypothalamus, and its primary role is to stimulate the anterior pituitary gland to secrete thyroid-stimulating hormone (TSH). TSH, in turn, acts on the thyroid gland, which prompts the production and release of the thyroid hormones T3 (triiodothyronine) and T4 (thyroxine), which are essential for the regulation of metabolism, growth, and energy balance. In clinical practice, synthetic TRH has been used to assess pituitary function during a TRH stimulation test. This diagnostic approach helps evaluate the integrity of the hypothalamic-pituitary-thyroid (HPT) axis, which identifies conditions such as secondary hypothyroidism or other pituitary dysfunctions.

Beyond diagnostics, research into TRH analogs has opened up potential therapeutic applications. Natural TRH has a relatively short half-life, which limits its direct clinical use. However, through structural modifications, such as peptide cyclization and the incorporation of non-natural amino acids, researchers have developed analogs with enhanced stability and prolonged activity. These analogs can more effectively modulate TSH release and, consequently, thyroid hormone synthesis. Recent studies, as highlighted in historical reviews of peptide hormone development, have shown promising results for TRH analogs in the management of thyroid dysfunction and even in certain neurodegenerative conditions where TRH's neuromodulatory roles may be beneficial.

Nursing Implications

- Monitor thyroid function through regular assessment of TSH, T3, and T4 levels, especially after TRH stimulation tests.
- Observe for clinical signs of thyroid dysfunction, such as changes in energy, weight, temperature sensitivity, or mood.
- Ensure accurate dosing and administration of synthetic TRH or TRH analogs. Follow institutional protocols.
- Be alert for any adverse reactions related to peptide administration, such as injection site discomfort or allergic responses.
- Inform patients about the purpose of TRH testing and the role of TRH analogs in the diagnosis and potential treatment of thyroid dysfunction.

- Educate patients on the importance of adherence to follow-up appointments and laboratory tests to monitor treatment efficacy.
- Work closely with endocrinologists and other healthcare providers to tailor therapy based on diagnostic findings and clinical response.
- Document and communicate any observed changes in patient condition to ensure timely adjustments in treatment.

Corticotropin-Releasing Hormone (CRH) and Adrenal Regulation

CRH, another hypothalamic peptide, helps control the body's response to stress via the HPA axis. Upon secretion, CRH binds to receptors on the anterior pituitary, which triggers the release of ACTH. ACTH then stimulates the adrenal cortex to produce cortisol, a glucocorticoid that is essential for managing stress, modulating immune responses, and regulating metabolism.

In clinical settings, synthetic CRH is often utilized in the CRH stimulation test, which helps diagnose disorders such as Cushing's syndrome or adrenal insufficiency. When a known quantity of CRH is administered and the ACTH and cortisol responses are measured, clinicians can evaluate the responsiveness of the HPA axis and pinpoint dysregulations.

As with TRH, the natural CRH molecule is subject to rapid degradation in circulation. Advances in peptide chemistry have led to the development of CRH analogs with improved stability and receptor selectivity. These modified peptides not only provide enhanced diagnostic precision but also present potential therapeutic avenues. For instance, in conditions characterized by hypercortisolism, such as Cushing's syndrome, CRH analogs might be employed to recalibrate cortisol production. Research continues to investigate the efficacy of these analogs in the modulation of cortisol levels and the potential alleviation of symptoms associated with chronic stress and adrenal disorders.

Integrate Research and Clinical Advances

The evolution of peptide hormone research over the past century, from the isolation of natural peptides to the synthesis of highly refined analogs, has significantly advanced our knowledge of endocrine regulation. Reviews such as those in *Peptide Hormones in Medicine: A 100-Year History* provide a comprehensive backdrop for these developments, which underscores how targeted modifications have overcome limitations like short half-lives and immunogenicity.

Moreover, modern textbooks illustrate the foundational biology of these peptide systems. They detail how the HPA axes coordinate endocrine functions. In the case of thyroid and adrenal health, the integration of these educational insights with cutting-edge biochemical research has led to the creation of peptide analogs that are not only more stable but also finely tuned to the physiological needs of individual patients.

Other Peptide Modulators

Advances in peptide engineering have led to the development of novel analogs that provide enhanced receptor specificity and improved pharmacokinetics. For instance, peptides that target receptors on thyroid and adrenal cells are being explored for their potential to fine-tune hormone output without the risk of overstimulation or suppression. Such targeted therapies could benefit patients with autoimmune thyroid disorders or adrenal insufficiency by providing a more balanced hormonal environment.

The delicate balance maintained by the thyroid and adrenal axes underscores the importance of precise hormonal regulation. Peptide-based approaches, with their inherent specificity and capacity for modification, provide a possible route to restore this balance in patients with endocrine dysfunctions.

Emergent Therapies for Hormonal-Related Disorders

In recent years, the field of peptide therapeutics has witnessed rapid advancements driven by innovations in molecular biology, high-throughput screening, and peptide synthesis. These developments have given rise to a new generation of peptide-based drugs that are not only more potent but also exhibit improved stability and bioavailability.

Engineered Peptide Analogs and Extended Half-Lives

One of the key challenges with natural peptides is their short half-life due to rapid degradation by peptidases. Through chemical modifications such as pegylation, cyclization, and incorporation of non-natural amino acids, researchers have been able to extend the half-life of these molecules without compromising their biological activity. Extended half-life peptides reduce the frequency of administration and improve patient compliance, which is particularly beneficial in chronic conditions like diabetes, GH deficiency, and thyroid disorders.

Multifunctional Peptides and Dual-Action Therapeutics

Emergent therapies are increasingly focused on peptides that can target multiple pathways simultaneously. For example, novel analogs are being developed to not only stimulate insulin secretion but also improve insulin sensitivity and reduce inflammation. Such multifunctional peptides could revolutionize the treatment of metabolic syndrome, where multiple hormonal imbalances contribute to disease pathology. Similarly, peptides that can modulate both the hypothalamic-pituitary-thyroid and hypothalamic-pituitary-adrenal axes are under investigation for complex endocrine disorders where overlapping dysfunctions occur.

Personalized Medicine and Peptide Therapies

The era of personalized medicine has influenced the development of peptide therapeutics. With advances in genomics and proteomics, it is now possible to tailor peptide treatments to an individual's specific hormonal profile and genetic makeup. This personalized approach ensures that therapies are not only more effective but also minimize the risk of adverse effects. For instance, patients with certain genetic predispositions may benefit from customized peptide analogs that are optimized for their receptor variants.

Novel Delivery Systems and Administration Routes

Another frontier in peptide therapeutics is the development of innovative delivery systems. Although many peptide drugs require subcutaneous or intramuscular injections, novel delivery mechanisms, including transdermal patches, nasal sprays, and oral formulations, are being actively researched. These new delivery routes could overcome one of the major limitations of peptide therapy—poor peroral bioavailability—which would expand the range of clinical applications and improve patient adherence.

Taken together, these emergent therapies underscore the dynamic nature of peptide research. When traditional knowledge of hormonal physiology is combined with cutting-edge biotechnology, researchers are poised to develop next-generation peptide drugs that address not only traditional endocrine disorders but also the complex, multifactorial conditions seen in modern metabolic diseases.

Side Effects During Peptide Therapy

Common Side Effects

Some of the most frequently encountered side effects during peptide therapy include injection site reactions, such as redness, swelling, discomfort and localized inflammation. Because peptides are proteins, there is also a risk of immunogenic responses, especially with repeated exposure or when non-native analogs are used. In some cases, patients may experience systemic side effects like nausea, headache, or alterations in appetite. For example, therapies that stimulate GH release can occasionally cause joint pain or water retention, while GLP-1 analogs might lead to gastrointestinal disturbances.

Strategies to Minimize Adverse Effects

To minimize these risks, modern peptide therapies often incorporate chemical modifications that reduce immunogenicity and prolong half-life without compromising activity. Dosing regimens are carefully titrated. Additionally, the use of controlled-release formulations and novel delivery systems helps mitigate peaks in concentration that might otherwise trigger side effects.

Monitor and Follow Up

Effective monitoring during peptide therapy is critical to ensure long-term safety and efficacy. Regular assessments of hormone levels (such as GH, insulin, TSH, or cortisol, based on the therapy) are essential to gauge the body's response. In patients who are treated for metabolic disorders, monitor blood glucose levels, lipid profiles, and body weight to provide important feedback on the therapy's impact. For those who receive peptide treatments for thyroid or adrenal dysfunction, periodic evaluations of thyroid function tests or adrenal axis studies are recommended.

Beyond biochemical monitoring, clinicians also pay close attention to clinical symptoms. Patient-reported outcomes, such as changes in energy levels, mood, or gastrointestinal function, are valuable to adjust dosage and frequency. In some cases, imaging studies or specialized functional tests may be employed to assess organ-specific effects, particularly when therapies are used off-label or in experimental settings.

Nursing Implications

- Inform patients about common side effects of peptide therapies, such as injection site reactions, localized inflammation, and potential systemic effects (nausea, headache, appetite changes).
- Educate patients on why they should report any unexpected or worsening symptoms, including signs of immunogenic reactions.
- Ensure proper administration techniques to minimize local reactions and maintain medication integrity.
- Follow titrated dosing regimens closely, particularly when treatment is started at a lower dose and gradually increased to a therapeutic level.
- Conduct frequent assessments of hormone levels (e.g., GH, insulin, TSH, cortisol) and other relevant

biochemical markers to evaluate therapeutic response.

- Monitor vital signs, weight, and patient-reported outcomes such as changes in energy levels, mood, and gastrointestinal function.
- Accurately document any adverse effects, patient responses, and changes in clinical status.
- Schedule regular follow-ups and coordinate with the healthcare team to adjust therapy as needed based on clinical and laboratory findings.
- Work closely with endocrinologists, pharmacists, and other healthcare professionals to ensure that peptide therapies are effectively tailored to individual patient needs.
- Utilize imaging studies or specialized tests when indicated, particularly in cases of off-label or experimental peptide use.

Chapter 7: Peptides in Cosmetics

The demand for scientifically advanced skin care has led to the rise of peptides as one of the most effective cosmetic ingredients. Peptides serve as fundamental building blocks of proteins such as collagen, elastin, and keratin. These proteins are essential to maintain skin structure, elasticity, and hydration. Unlike traditional skin care ingredients, peptides provide targeted benefits because they stimulate the biological pathways involved in skin repair and rejuvenation.

With age, exposure to ultraviolet radiation, pollution, and oxidative stress, the skin's natural production of collagen and elastin declines, which causes wrinkles, sagging, and uneven skin tone. Peptides counteract these effects because they promote collagen synthesis, inhibit muscle contractions responsible for expression lines, and regulate melanin production to improve pigmentation issues.

Mechanisms of Peptides in Skin Rejuvenation

Peptides play a pivotal role in modern skin care. They provide targeted benefits that enhance skin rejuvenation, improve texture, and combat aging. These short chains of amino acids serve as biochemical messengers that influence cellular activity, stimulate protein synthesis, and regulate various physiological processes in the skin. Through the integration of peptides into cosmetic formulations, researchers and skin care professionals have developed advanced products that support skin homeostasis and resilience.

Peptides exert their effects through several biological mechanisms, categorized into four primary groups: signal peptides, carrier peptides, neurotransmitter-inhibitory peptides, and enzyme-inhibitory peptides. Each category has a unique function that contributes to skin repair, hydration, elasticity, and overall appearance.

Signal Peptides

Signal peptides act as cellular messengers. They direct fibroblasts to produce essential components of the extracellular matrix, such as collagen, elastin, and glycosaminoglycans. These peptides mimic natural growth factors and trigger regenerative processes that help maintain skin firmness and elasticity. Their function is particularly critical in anti-aging skin care, as they work to reduce the appearance of fine lines and wrinkles.

Examples:

- **Palmitoyl Pentapeptide-4 (Matrixyl 3000):** Matrixyl 3000 is a peptide complex that contains Palmitoyl Tripeptide-1 and Palmitoyl Tetrapeptide-7, which together stimulate fibroblast activity, increase collagen production, and reduce signs of aging, including fine lines and sagging skin. It is widely used in anti-aging formulations to enhance skin texture and resilience.
- **Palmitoyl Tripeptide-5:** Palmitoyl Tripeptide-5 stimulates collagen production by interacting with transforming growth factor-beta (TGF-β) receptors, improving skin structure and reducing wrinkle depth. This mechanism contributes to improved

skin structure, reduced wrinkle depth and increased skin smoothness over time.

Carrier Peptides

Carrier peptides facilitate the transport of essential minerals such as copper and manganese into skin cells. These minerals are vital for enzymatic reactions that drive collagen synthesis, wound healing, and antioxidant defense mechanisms. Because they deliver these trace elements directly to the skin, carrier peptides accelerate tissue repair and improve overall skin vitality.

- **GHK-Cu (Copper Tripeptide-1):** A well-researched peptide that binds to copper ions, promotes wound healing, reduces inflammation, and stimulates the production of collagen and elastin. This peptide reverses visible signs of aging and improves skin tone and texture.
- **Manganese Tripeptide-1:** This peptide enhances the skin's antioxidant defenses and protects against oxidative stress and environmental damage. It supports collagen biosynthesis for firmer, healthier skin.

Neurotransmitter-Inhibitory Peptides

Neurotransmitter-inhibitory peptides, often referred to as "Botox-like" peptides, target muscle contractions that lead to expression lines and dynamic wrinkles. These peptides modulate neuromuscular communication because they inhibit neurotransmitter release, effectively reduce the movement of facial muscles and prevent the formation of deep wrinkles over time.

Examples:

- **Acetyl Hexapeptide-8 (Argireline):** This widely used peptide interferes with the SNARE complex. It blocks the release of acetylcholine, a neurotransmitter responsible for muscle contraction. Because it relaxes facial muscles, Argireline helps to diminish fine lines and prevent wrinkle formation.
- **Pentapeptide-18:** This peptide inhibits calcium influx in neuronal cells, reduces muscle contractions and helps smooth dynamic wrinkles around the forehead and eyes. It provides a muscle-relaxant effect and maintains natural facial expressions. It helps smooth out dynamic wrinkles around the forehead and eyes but doesn't alter facial mobility significantly.

Enzyme-Inhibitory Peptides

Enzyme-inhibitory peptides protect the skin because they prevent the degradation of collagen, elastin, and hyaluronic acid. These peptides block matrix metalloproteinases (MMPs) enzymes that break down structural proteins and contribute to skin aging. Because they inhibit these enzymes, peptides help maintain skin integrity, hydration, and elasticity.

Examples:

- **Rice-Derived Peptides:** These peptides reduce MMP activity and simultaneously stimulate hyaluronic acid synthesis, which results in improved skin hydration and elasticity. They are commonly used in anti-aging and moisturizing formulations.

- **Soy Oligopeptides:** With anti-inflammatory and antioxidant properties, soy-derived peptides protect against environmental stressors, including ultraviolet radiation and pollution. Because they neutralize free radicals and reduce collagen degradation, they help maintain youthful skin.

Popular Cosmetic Peptides

Peptides are widely incorporated into serums, creams, masks, and other skin care formulations because they provide targeted solutions that enhance skin rejuvenation. Below are some of the most well-known cosmetic peptides and their applications in modern skin care.

Matrixyl 3000 (Palmitoyl Tripeptide-1 + Palmitoyl Tetrapeptide-7)

Matrixyl 3000 is one of the most well-researched anti-aging peptides. It's known for its ability to stimulate collagen production, improve skin hydration, and reduce the appearance of wrinkles. Because it mimics the natural signaling mechanisms of the skin, this peptide complex enhances elasticity and firmness, which makes it a popular ingredient in anti-aging formulations.

Usage in Modern Cosmetics

- Commonly found in anti-aging creams, serums, and moisturizers.

- Helps improve overall skin texture and elasticity.

- Works well in combination with hyaluronic acid and antioxidants for enhanced hydration and skin repair.

Nursing Implications

- Nurses and skin care professionals should educate patients on the benefits of using Matrixyl 3000 for long-term anti-aging effects.
- Matrixyl 3000 is well-tolerated by most skin types, but individuals with sensitive skin should perform a patch test before use.
- Encourage patients to use complementary skin care products such as broad-spectrum sunscreen. This will maximize the anti-aging benefits of Matrixyl 3000.

Syn-Ake (Dipeptide Diaminobutyroyl Benzylamide Diacetate)

Syn-Ake is a synthetic peptide designed to mimic the muscle-relaxant effects of snake venom. Because it inhibits muscle contractions, it reduces the formation of dynamic wrinkles, particularly on the forehead and around the eyes.

Usage in Modern Cosmetics

- Commonly incorporated into anti-aging serums and creams targeting fine lines and expression wrinkles.

- Often used as a non-invasive alternative to Botox, it provides a temporary muscle-relaxing effect without injections.
- Works well in formulations with hydrating agents like glycerin and peptides that support collagen production.

Nursing Implications

- Nurses should inform patients that while Syn-Ake can help smooth expression lines, its effects are temporary and require consistent use for visible results.
- Educate patients on potential contraindications for individuals with certain skin conditions or hypersensitivity to synthetic peptides.
- Emphasize the importance of Syn-Ake used in combination with sunscreen to prevent UV-induced collagen degradation.

Tetrapeptide-30

Tetrapeptide-30 helps regulate tyrosinase activity, which has a role in melanin production as it reduces hyperpigmentation and promotes a more even skin tone. It reduces hyperpigmentation, dark spots, and uneven skin tone.

Usage in Modern Cosmetics

- Found in brightening and anti-pigmentation creams and serums.

- Often combined with ingredients like niacinamide, vitamin C, and alpha-arbutin for enhanced skin-lightening effects.
- Used in formulations that target melasma, post-inflammatory hyperpigmentation, and sunspots.

Nursing Implications

- Nurses should educate patients on the gradual effects of Tetrapeptide-30, as pigmentation correction takes time.
- Recommend daily sunscreen application to prevent further hyperpigmentation while using brightening treatments.
- Advise individuals with sensitive skin to introduce these peptides gradually to avoid irritation.

Tripeptide-10 Citrulline

This peptide regulates collagen fiber organization, which improves skin firmness and texture. It helps optimize the skin's extracellular matrix, which makes the skin appear more youthful and resilient.

Usage in Modern Cosmetics

- Found in anti-aging creams and firming serums that promote skin elasticity.
- Works well in conjunction with peptides that boost collagen and antioxidants to support skin integrity.

- Often included in high-end skin care formulations designed for mature skin.

<u>Nursing Implications</u>

- Inform patients that Tripeptide-10 Citrulline works best with consistent application and other collagen-supporting skin care ingredients.
- Encourage hydration and a nutrient-rich diet to support collagen production naturally.
- Remind patients that collagen degradation is influenced by lifestyle factors such as smoking, poor diet, and UV exposure.

The Role of Peptides in Modern Skin Care

Peptides have revolutionized modern skin care because they provide targeted solutions for anti-aging, hydration, brightening, and skin repair. Due to advancements in cosmetic science, peptides are now formulated into various skin care products, including serums, masks, and moisturizers. Their ability to deliver results without invasive procedures makes them popular among dermatologists, skin care professionals, and consumers alike.

Nursing Considerations in Peptide-Based Skin Care

As the demand for peptide-based skin care grows, nurses and skin care specialists play a vital role in patient education and product recommendations. When they advise patients on peptide-based skin care, they should:

- Assess individual skin concerns to recommend the most appropriate peptide formulations.
- Highlight the importance of consistent use for visible results.
- Educate patients on the use of peptides combined with complementary skin care (e.g., antioxidants, sunscreen, and moisturizers) to enhance effectiveness.
- Encourage patients to perform a patch test before they incorporate new peptides into their routine.

Peptides in Collagen Production and Wrinkle Reduction

Collagen loss is a primary factor in skin aging, which causes wrinkles, sagging, and loss of elasticity. Peptides stimulate collagen production, prevent collagen breakdown, and enhance skin hydration. Their targeted action makes them a key component in both medical and cosmetic dermatology.

Stimulate Collagen Biosynthesis

Signal peptides act as biological messengers that activate fibroblasts to produce more collagen, elastin, and glycosaminoglycans. This results in improved skin firmness and reduced wrinkle formation over time.

Prevent Collagen Breakdown

Aging and environmental factors such as UV exposure and pollution lead to increased activity of MMPs, enzymes that degrade collagen and elastin. Enzyme-inhibitory peptides counteract this degradation, which helps maintain skin structure and prevent premature aging.

- **Tetrapeptide-21** – Supports collagen synthesis and skin repair, as it helps to improve skin elasticity and resilience.

Enhance Skin Hydration

Hydration is essential to maintain skin elasticity and prevent fine lines. Carrier peptides transport trace elements like copper and manganese, which are necessary for enzymatic processes involved in skin repair and hydration.

Clinical and Cosmetological Implications

Clinical Implications

- **Dermatology & Anti-Aging Treatments** – Peptides are widely used in clinical dermatology to manage premature aging, post-procedure recovery, and wound healing due to their regenerative properties.

- **Scar Reduction Therapy** – Copper peptides and signal peptides are commonly included in scar treatment regimens to promote tissue repair and collagen deposition.

- **Post-Invasive Procedures** – Peptide-infused skin care is frequently recommended after chemical peels, laser treatments, and microneedling to accelerate healing and minimize inflammation.

Cosmetological Implications

- **Anti-Wrinkle Formulations** – Peptides are key ingredients in anti-aging serums and creams that target fine lines, deep wrinkles, and skin firmness.
- **Professional Skin Care Treatments** – Many high-end facials and mesotherapy procedures incorporate peptide-based serums for enhanced skin rejuvenation.
- **Combination Therapy** – Peptides work synergistically with hyaluronic acid, retinoids, and vitamin C to maximize collagen synthesis and hydration.
- **Safe Alternative to Botox** – Neurotransmitter-inhibitory peptides, such as Argireline (Acetyl Hexapeptide-3), provide a Botox-like effect because they relax facial muscles and reduce expression wrinkles without injections.

Peptides Target Pigmentation and Skin Tone

Uneven pigmentation and dark spots result from excessive melanin production, often triggered by factors such as sun exposure, inflammation, hormonal changes, and aging. Peptides regulate melanogenesis because they either inhibit tyrosinase activity, block melanin transport, or modulate melanocyte-stimulating hormone (α-MSH) signaling. These mechanisms make peptide-based treatments effective to treat hyperpigmentation, melasma, and post-inflammatory discoloration.

Key Peptides for Pigmentation Control

Decapeptide-12

- A potent tyrosinase inhibitor that prevents the overproduction of melanin.
- Commonly used in clinical treatments for melasma, age spots, and post-inflammatory hyperpigmentation.
- Studies suggest that Decapeptide-12 can significantly reduce pigmentation in as little as four weeks of consistent application.

Acetyl Hexapeptide-1

- Modulates the α-MSH pathway, which helps to balance pigmentation and reduce hyperpigmentation, but it does not directly prevent hypopigmentation.
- Helps restore even skin tone and is beneficial for those with vitiligo or pigmentation disorders.
- Also provides anti-inflammatory benefits, which makes it suitable for sensitive skin types.

Nonapeptide-1

- Inhibits melanin production because it blocks the activation of key enzymes responsible for melanogenesis.

- Effectively reduces post-inflammatory hyperpigmentation caused by acne, laser treatments, or sun exposure.
- Often included in brightening serums and creams to even out skin tone gradually.

Peptide-Based Brightening Treatments vs. Traditional Ingredients

Peptide-based brightening treatments are safer and more skin-friendly alternatives to traditional depigmenting agents such as hydroquinone, which has been linked to long-term skin sensitivity, irritation, and potential cytotoxicity. Unlike hydroquinone, peptides provide targeted action without disruption to overall skin health.

Clinical and Cosmetological Implications

Clinical Applications

- Used in dermatological treatments for melasma, sunspots, and post-inflammatory hyperpigmentation.
- Recommended for post-laser and chemical peel recovery to prevent rebound pigmentation.
- Incorporated into prescription and medical-grade skin care formulations to provide gradual but long-term improvements in skin tone.

Cosmetological Applications

- Featured in brightening serums, spot treatments, and daily moisturizers to promote radiant and even-toned skin.
- Popular in anti-aging skin care regimens, as uneven pigmentation is a key contributor to an aged appearance.
- Frequently combined with Vitamin C, niacinamide, and exfoliating acids for enhanced skin-brightening effects.

Innovations in Peptide Delivery Systems

Peptides are highly effective bioactive compounds in skin care, but their large molecular weight and hydrophilic nature pose challenges for skin penetration. Without proper delivery methods, peptides may not reach the deeper layers of the skin, which limits their efficacy. Advances in cosmetic science have led to innovative delivery systems that enhance bioavailability, stability, and targeted absorption of peptides, which ensures maximum skin care benefits.

Peptide-Infused Creams

Creams provide an excellent medium for long-term hydration and sustained peptide delivery. Innovations in cream-based peptide formulations include:

- **Encapsulated Peptides in Liposomes & Niosomes**: Protect peptides from oxidation and degradation. Enhance penetration into deeper layers of the epidermis. Allow for slow, controlled release, which ensures prolonged skin benefits.

- **Multi-Peptide Complexes:** Combine different peptides (e.g., signal peptides, carrier peptides) to provide comprehensive anti-aging effects. Improve skin elasticity, hydration, and firmness.

- **Nanocarrier Systems**: Utilize solid lipid nanoparticles and nano-emulsions to enhance peptide stability. Ensure better skin absorption but may alter the skin barrier function depending on the formulation.

Advanced Peptide Serums

Serums are lightweight formulations that deliver high concentrations of active peptides directly into the skin. Innovations in peptide serums include:

- **Microemulsion Technology:** Creates ultra-fine particles for superior penetration and bioavailability. Ensures even distribution of peptides across the skin surface.

- **Hydrogel and Biopolymer-Based Serums:** Contain hyaluronic acid or alginate matrices to improve peptide hydration and absorption. Provide long-term effects because they form a moisture-retentive barrier on the skin.

- **Combination with Penetration Enhancers:** Peptide serums now include carrier molecules such as phospholipids or penetration enhancers like niacinamide to facilitate deeper absorption.

Synergistic blends with antioxidants (e.g., Vitamin C, resveratrol) enhance skin renewal and protect from oxidative damage.

Clinical and Consumer Benefits

The advancements in peptide creams and serums provide both clinical and consumer benefits.

- **Enhanced Anti-Aging Effects:** Peptides in optimized formulations provide faster wrinkle reduction, improved hydration, and increased collagen production.

- **Gentle and Non-Irritating:** Unlike traditional anti-aging ingredients like retinoids, peptide-based skin care is well-tolerated and suitable for sensitive skin.

- **Sustained and Targeted Delivery:** Controlled-release mechanisms ensure peptides are continuously active, which causes prolonged skin benefits.

- **Customization for Specific Concerns:** Innovations allow for the development of targeted peptide creams and serums for concerns like hyperpigmentation, redness, and loss of firmness.

Nursing Implications

As the use of peptides in dermatology grows, nursing professionals must be aware of their role in skin health, wound healing, and cosmetic procedures.

Patient Education on Peptide Efficacy

Nurses should educate patients on how peptides work, their benefits, and proper application methods to maximize results. Patients should be informed about the importance of consistent use, as peptide treatments often require long-term application for visible improvements.

Pre- and Post-Treatment Care for Advanced Peptide Delivery

- **Microneedling & Iontophoresis**: Nurses prepare patients for these procedures and ensure proper skin cleansing and post-procedure care to minimize irritation and maximize results.
- **Topical Peptide Therapy**: In clinical settings, nurses may help apply peptide-based treatments, especially in post-laser recovery, wound healing, and scar reduction.

Monitor for Adverse Reactions

- Although peptides are generally well-tolerated, patients with sensitive skin may experience mild irritation or allergic reactions.
- Nurses should be aware of potential interactions with other skin care treatments and advise patients accordingly.

Comparative Effectiveness with Traditional Skin Care Ingredients

Peptides vs. Retinoids

Retinoids, derived from vitamin A, are widely recognized for their powerful anti-aging properties. They stimulate collagen production, accelerate cell turnover, and reduce the appearance of fine lines and wrinkles. However, retinoids can often lead to skin irritation, redness, and peeling, particularly during the initial stages of use. This is due to their potent exfoliation properties, which can disrupt the skin's natural barrier, especially for individuals with sensitive skin.

Peptides, on the other hand, provide a gentler approach. Peptides help to stimulate collagen production and enhance the skin's barrier function. Unlike retinoids, they are less likely to irritate, which makes them a better choice for people with sensitive skin or those who want to avoid the redness and peeling often associated with retinoid use. Even though peptides may take longer to show visible results compared to the faster exfoliating effects of retinoids, they provide a sustainable and less irritating option for long-term anti-aging benefits.

Peptides vs. Antioxidants

Antioxidants, such as vitamins C and E, protect the skin from oxidative stress caused by free radicals, which are unstable molecules that contribute to premature aging. Because they neutralize these free radicals, antioxidants help to protect the skin from environmental damage, such as pollution and UV radiation, which prevents fine lines, wrinkles, and hyperpigmentation.

Even though antioxidants are essential for skin health, peptides provide a more targeted and active role in skin renewal. Although antioxidants mainly protect against oxidative stress, peptides contribute to both protection and active skin renewal by stimulating collagen production and cell repair. For instance, peptides can enhance collagen production, promote cell turnover, and improve skin texture, which addresses not only the signs of aging but also the skin's overall function. This makes peptides an essential ingredient for skin rejuvenation. They work at a deeper cellular level than antioxidants, which are more focused on protection than active stimulation.

Peptides vs. Hyaluronic Acid

Hyaluronic acid is renowned for its ability to retain moisture and provide immediate plumping effects to the skin. Because it draws water into the skin, it helps to improve hydration and smooth out fine lines. It is commonly used in moisturizers, serums, and dermal fillers to provide a temporary youthful glow and improve skin elasticity.

Peptides and hyaluronic acid complement each other beautifully. Although hyaluronic acid hydrates and plumps the skin, peptides work on a cellular level to stimulate the production of collagen and elastin, key proteins responsible for the skin's firmness and elasticity. When these two ingredients are combined, skin care products can provide both immediate hydration and long-term structural improvements. The synergy between peptides and hyaluronic acid enhances the skin's ability to maintain moisture and improves its overall elasticity, which causes smoother, more youthful skin over time.

One of the most significant benefits of peptides over some traditional skin care ingredients is their suitability for long-term use, as they usually do not cause irritation or compromise the skin barrier. Retinoids, for example, may produce visible changes in skin texture and tone relatively quickly, but they come with the downside of potential irritation and peeling. This can make continued use difficult, especially for those with sensitive skin. Over time, this can also diminish the skin's tolerance to the ingredient, which requires adjustments in the routine.

Peptides, in contrast, provide a more balanced and gradual approach to anti-aging. Because they support the skin's natural functions, such as collagen production, cell turnover, and hydration, peptides provide long-term improvements without harsh side effects. They support the skin's health over time and promote a more youthful and resilient complexion without the need for frequent breaks or adjustments. Peptides' ability to strengthen the skin barrier and boost its natural renewal process makes them a sustainable anti-aging solution that works in harmony with the skin's natural rhythm.

Peptides in Combination with Traditional Skin Care Ingredients

One of the key advantages of peptides is their versatility and compatibility with other ingredients. Peptides enhance skin care ingredients' effectiveness when used together. For instance:

- **With Retinoids**: Even though retinoids can be irritants, when they're combined with peptides, this can help mitigate some of the dryness and redness. Peptides work to support the skin's barrier, which helps to reduce irritation and enhance the benefits of retinoids.

- **With Antioxidants**: Use of peptides alongside antioxidants provides a double layer of protection and rejuvenation. Antioxidants protect the skin from free radicals, while peptides stimulate the skin's natural repair and regeneration processes, which causes healthier, more youthful skin.

- **With Hyaluronic Acid**: As mentioned earlier, peptides and hyaluronic acid work synergistically to address both hydration and skin structure. Though hyaluronic acid delivers instant plumping effects, peptides work to improve skin elasticity and firmness over time, which causes a more comprehensive anti-aging approach.

Chapter 8: Peptides for Sexual Health

Peptides' potential to enhance sexual health has garnered significant attention in recent years.

Mechanism of Peptides in Sexual Function Improvement

Peptides help improve sexual function because they target different physiological processes, such as neurotransmitter regulation, hormonal balance, and vascular function. These mechanisms help address common sexual dysfunction, including low libido, erectile dysfunction (ED), and female sexual arousal disorder (FSAD). Below is an in-depth look at how peptides influence these key areas.

Neurotransmitter Modulation

Neurotransmitters in the brain play a critical role in the regulation of sexual desire and arousal. Peptides interact with these neurotransmitters and modulate neural pathways that are essential for sexual behavior.

- **Kisspeptin:** Kisspeptin is a neuropeptide that has emerged as a key regulator of sexual behavior, particularly in women. It stimulates the release of gonadotropin-releasing hormone (GnRH), which then triggers the release of reproductive hormones like luteinizing hormone (LH) and follicle-stimulating hormone (FSH). Studies have shown that kisspeptin can enhance sexual desire and behavior because it activates specific brain regions involved in sexual arousal. In both men and women, the stimulation of kisspeptin receptors in the hypothalamus is associated with increased sexual motivation and arousal, although its role in orgasmic response remains under investigation. This makes kisspeptin a candidate for therapeutic interventions for those with hypoactive sexual desire disorder (HSDD) and other sexual dysfunctions.

- **PT-141 (Bremelanotide):** Bremelanotide is another peptide that exerts its effects through the nervous system, although it operates differently from kisspeptin. PT-141 primarily binds to melanocortin receptors MC3 and MC4 in the brain, which are involved in the regulation of sexual desire and arousal. These receptors are involved in the regulation of sexual desire and arousal. Because it stimulates melanocortin receptors, PT-141 activates neural pathways that lead to increased sexual desire in both men and women. Unlike traditional treatments for sexual dysfunction, such as sildenafil (Viagra), which work through the vascular system, PT-141 directly targets the brain's sexual centers, which makes it an effective option for people with sexual arousal disorders.

The modulation of neurotransmitters by these peptides results in the enhancement of sexual desire, improved arousal, and an increase in overall sexual satisfaction.

Hormonal Regulation

Peptides also influence hormonal levels that are integral to sexual function. Hormones control various aspects of reproductive health, including libido, sexual performance, and fertility. Through hormonal regulation, peptides can help restore balance and improve sexual function.

- **Bremelanotide (PT-141):** Although mainly known for its role in the activation of melanocortin receptors, PT-141 also affects hormonal regulation in the brain. The peptide has been shown to influence the release of dopamine, a neurotransmitter critical for sexual motivation and arousal. The regulation of dopamine levels by PT-141 can enhance sexual desire, which makes it a valuable treatment for people who suffer from low libido or sexual arousal issues. Unlike other therapies that focus solely on the vascular system, PT-141 directly affects the neural mechanisms that underlie sexual motivation, which provides a new and effective avenue for treatment.

- **Kisspeptin:** As a powerful regulator of reproductive hormones, kisspeptin has a significant impact on hormonal balance. Because it promotes the release of GnRH, kisspeptin indirectly stimulates the secretion of LH and FSH, which are critical for the menstrual cycle and fertility. Kisspeptin indirectly influences the production of estrogen and progesterone by stimulating GnRH release, which regulates the secretion of LH and FSH in the pituitary gland. In men, kisspeptin's ability to modulate testosterone levels can improve libido and sexual function. This hormonal regulation is essential for sexual health, especially in individuals with hormonal imbalances.

The hormonal effects of peptides not only regulate sexual function but also help manage conditions such as ED, low libido, and sexual arousal disorders.

Vascular Effects

Blood flow to the sexual organs is a critical determinant of sexual performance. In men, erectile function relies on adequate blood supply to the penis, while in women, increased blood flow to the clitoris and vaginal tissues enhances sexual arousal. Certain peptides have vasodilatory effects, which promote blood circulation and improve sexual function.

- **PT-141 (Bremelanotide):** One of the most notable aspects of PT-141's mechanism is its ability to enhance blood flow to sexual organs. Although it mainly affects the nervous system, PT-141 also has a mild vasodilatory effect. This improvement in blood circulation can enhance erectile function in men and sexual arousal in women, especially when the primary issue is related to arousal rather than desire. In women, for example, PT-141 increases blood flow to the genital area, which improves sensitivity and sexual satisfaction. The peptide has been found to have a direct impact on the vascular response during sexual arousal, which makes it an effective treatment for both men and women with sexual dysfunction.

- **Other Peptides with Vascular Effects:** Apomorphine, a dopamine receptor agonist, improves sexual function mainly through central nervous system activation rather than direct vasodilatory effects. Apomorphine is a dopamine agonist that increases blood flow to the penis, which improves erectile function. Although not as widely used as PT-141, Apomorphine has shown promise in the treatment of ED because it targets the vascular system and improves blood circulation.

Peptides that improve blood flow can significantly enhance sexual performance because they address one of the fundamental physiological requirements for sexual activity—an adequate blood supply to the sexual organs.

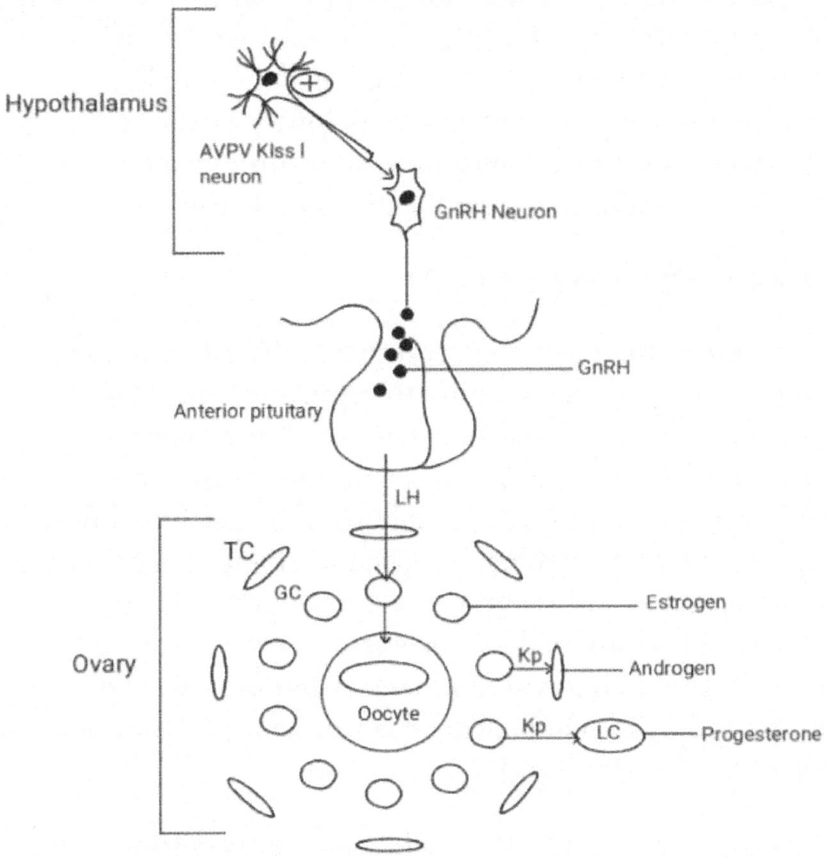

Fig 13: Mechanism of action of Kisspeptin

Roles Peptides Play in the Treatment of Erectile Dysfunction and Female Arousal Disorders

Peptides, particularly PT-141, have emerged as treatments for sexual dysfunction, particularly in the areas of ED and female arousal disorders. Unlike traditional medications that focus mainly on the vascular mechanisms involved in sexual function, PT-141 provides a novel approach because it targets the nervous system. This mechanism of action provides an alternative or adjunctive therapy for individuals who experience sexual dysfunction due to neural or hormonal imbalances. Below, we explore PT-141's role in ED and female arousal disorders, along with the clinical and nursing implications of its use.

Erectile Dysfunction (ED)

ED is one of the most common sexual disorders in men, characterized by the inability to achieve or maintain an erection sufficient for sexual activity. Traditional treatments for ED, such as phosphodiesterase type 5 inhibitors (e.g., sildenafil, tadalafil), improve blood flow to the penis, which enables the vascular changes necessary for an erection. However, these medications may not be effective for all individuals, particularly those whose ED is not solely related to vascular causes but may also be influenced by psychological or neurological factors. This is where PT-141 stands out.

PT-141 primarily activates melanocortin receptors in the brain, specifically MC3 and MC4 receptors, which are involved in sexual arousal and desire. This peptide bypasses the vascular pathways targeted by traditional ED medications and instead stimulates the CNS, which directly influences sexual desire and arousal. PT-141 enhances the body's physiological response to sexual stimuli, which improves erectile function.

In clinical trials, PT-141 has been shown to effectively treat ED, particularly in men who do not respond to traditional medications. A study published in *The Journal of Sexual Medicine* demonstrated that PT-141 significantly improved erectile function and sexual satisfaction in men with ED. Importantly, PT-141 has been shown to have a relatively quick onset of action. Some patients experience improvements within hours of administration. Its effectiveness is attributed to the peptide's ability to enhance the sexual experience through neural pathways, which makes it an excellent alternative for men who do not respond to PDE5 inhibitors or those who experience side effects from these medications.

Nursing Implications

Nurses should assess the causes of erectile dysfunction in patients before they recommend PT-141, as the peptide may not be effective for all causes of ED, particularly when vascular health is significantly compromised. Nurses should educate patients on the potential side effects of PT-141, which may include mild nausea, headache, and flushing. It is also essential to discuss the appropriate administration of PT-141, which is usually through subcutaneous injection, and ensure patients are comfortable with this method of delivery.

Female Arousal Disorders

FSAD is characterized by a persistent or recurrent inability to achieve or maintain sexual arousal despite adequate sexual desire and stimulation. This condition often co-occurs with HSDD, where women experience a lack of sexual desire. HSDD and FSAD can be caused by a combination of hormonal imbalances, psychological factors, and neurological dysfunction. PT-141 targets the neural pathways responsible for sexual arousal.

Mechanism of Action in Female Arousal Disorders

Like in men, PT-141 enhances sexual arousal in women because it acts on melanocortin receptors in the brain. The peptide stimulates the CNS and increases sexual desire and arousal in response to sexual stimuli. This mechanism is particularly beneficial for women who experience arousal difficulties due to psychological or hormonal factors, such as stress, menopause, or hormonal contraceptive use. PT-141 has been shown to improve arousal, sexual satisfaction, and overall quality of sexual life.

Clinical Studies

In clinical trials, PT-141 has proven to be effective in the treatment of female sexual dysfunction, especially in premenopausal women with HSDD. A pivotal study published in *The Journal of Sexual Medicine* showed that women who received PT-141 injections experienced a significant increase in sexual desire and satisfaction compared to those who received a placebo. These effects were noted both in laboratory settings and in real-life situations. Women who had previously been unresponsive to oral therapies for sexual dysfunction, such as flibanserin, saw notable improvements with PT-141. This suggests its potential as a treatment option for those with more complex sexual dysfunctions.

Nursing Implications

Nurses who care for women with sexual arousal disorders should assess the emotional, psychological, and hormonal factors that may contribute to the patient's sexual difficulties. When PT-141 is considered a treatment option, it is essential to monitor for side effects, which may include mild headaches, flushing, and nausea. Nurses should also provide education about the administration of PT-141, which involves subcutaneous injection, and ensure that patients feel comfortable with the injection process. Additionally, nurses should be aware of the importance of an open, nonjudgmental communication channel to discuss sexual health concerns, as these issues may be sensitive for some patients.

Sexual health disorders can have significant psychological and emotional impacts on patients. Nurses should provide a supportive environment where patients can discuss their concerns and feelings. They should assess for any psychological conditions, such as depression or anxiety, that may contribute to sexual dysfunction and encourage patients to seek therapy if appropriate.

Sexual health is deeply connected to overall physical and mental well-being. Nurses should take a holistic approach when they manage sexual dysfunction and consider the role of hormones, psychological factors, and overall health. When they administer PT-141 or other peptide therapies, nurses should work in collaboration with other healthcare providers to ensure comprehensive care.

Nurses should monitor patients for any adverse reactions or changes in sexual function after starting PT-141 therapy. Follow-up visits are essential to assess the effectiveness of the treatment and to adjust the dosage or treatment plan if necessary. Nurses should also monitor for any contraindications or interactions with other medications, especially for patients on hormone therapy or medications for other chronic conditions.

Ethical and Safety Considerations

Although peptide therapy provides benefits, it is essential to consider ethical and safety aspects. Clinical studies have reported that PT-141 has a favorable safety profile, with most treatment-emergent adverse events being mild or moderate in intensity.

PT-141 (Bremelanotide) is approved by the FDA for the treatment of acquired, generalized hypoactive sexual desire disorder (HSDD) in premenopausal women. However, it is not approved for the treatment of sexual dysfunction in men or postmenopausal women.

The use of peptides in sexual health raises ethical questions about accessibility, informed consent, and the potential for misuse. Healthcare providers must ensure that patients are fully informed about the benefits and risks associated with peptide therapy.

Chapter 9: Peptides for Gut Health

The human gut is far more than just a digestive organ; it is a sophisticated ecosystem where digestion, nutrient absorption, and immune functions intersect. This intricate system is often called the "second brain." It is home to trillions of microorganisms, collectively known as the gut microbiome, which plays a pivotal role in maintaining overall health. When this delicate balance is disrupted, it can cause a host of gastrointestinal disorders, such as irritable bowel syndrome (IBS), inflammatory bowel disease (IBD), and leaky gut syndrome. The gut is a dynamic environment where food is broken down into nutrients, which are absorbed into the bloodstream to fuel the body. However, its functions extend far beyond digestion. The gut is also a critical immune system component that houses approximately seventy percent of the body's immune cells. This immune-gut connection defends against pathogens while maintaining tolerance to beneficial microbes and food antigens.

The gut microbiome is central to this process. It is composed of bacteria, viruses, fungi, and other microorganisms. A healthy microbiome aids digestion, produces essential vitamins (like vitamin K and some B vitamins), and helps regulate the immune system. However, imbalances in the microbiome (dysbiosis) can cause inflammation, impaired gut barrier function, and the development of chronic conditions such as IBS, IBD, and leaky gut syndrome.

In recent years, scientific research has highlighted the importance of peptides to support gut health. These tiny but mighty molecules have emerged as key players in digestion, gut lining repair, microbiome balance, and even the treatment of gut-related disorders.

Peptides have garnered significant attention for the following abilities related to gut health.

- **Aid Digestion:** Certain peptides, such as those derived from dietary proteins, act as bioactive compounds that stimulate digestive enzymes and improve nutrient absorption. For example, bioactive peptides from milk proteins (like casein and whey) have been shown to enhance the breakdown of food in the gut, which makes nutrients more accessible to the body.
- **Repair the Gut Lining:** The gut lining (epithelial barrier) is a single layer of cells that separates the gut lumen from the bloodstream. When this barrier is compromised, it is called leaky gut syndrome. This condition allows harmful substances like bacteria and toxins to enter the bloodstream, which triggers inflammation and immune responses. Peptides such as glutamine-rich peptides and collagen peptides promote epithelial cell regeneration and enhance the production of tight junction proteins. This action strengthens the gut lining and seals the gaps between cells.
- **Balance the Microbiome:** Peptides promote the growth of beneficial bacteria (probiotics) and inhibit the growth of harmful pathogens, which can modulate the composition of the gut microbiome. For instance, antimicrobial peptides (AMPs), which are naturally produced by the gut's epithelial cells,

help maintain microbial balance as they target and neutralize pathogenic bacteria.

- **Treat Gut Disorders:** Peptides are being explored as therapeutic agents for various gut disorders. For example, glucagon-like peptide-1 (GLP-1), a peptide hormone produced in the gut, has been shown to reduce inflammation and improve gut motility in patients with IBS. Similarly, teduglutide, a synthetic analog of GLP-2, treats short bowel syndrome by promoting intestinal growth and absorption.

Peptides and Digestion

Digestion is a highly intricate process that transforms food into absorbable nutrients that provide the body with the energy and the building blocks it needs to function. This process relies heavily on enzymatic activity, gut motility, and a balanced gut microbiome. Peptides play a dual role in digestion. They facilitate enzymatic breakdown and regulate gut function.

Digestion begins in the mouth and continues in the stomach and small intestine, where enzymes break down complex macronutrients—proteins, carbohydrates, and fats—into simpler forms that can be absorbed. Peptides derived from digestive enzymes play a critical role in this process, particularly in protein digestion.

Two key enzymes involved in protein digestion are Pepsin and Trypsin. Pepsin, secreted in the stomach, breaks down proteins into smaller peptides. Trypsin, produced in the pancreas and activated in the small intestine, further cleaves these peptides into individual amino acids. These amino acids are then absorbed through the intestinal lining and transported to cells throughout the body.

Beyond enzymatic breakdown, certain peptides act as bioactive molecules. For example, peptides derived from dietary proteins (such as casein in milk) have been shown to enhance the activity of digestive enzymes, which improves nutrient absorption efficiency.

Gut motility is the rhythmic contractions of the gastrointestinal (GI) tract that propel food and waste through the digestive system. Proper motility is essential for efficient digestion and prevents constipation, diarrhea, or bloating. Peptides help regulate gut motility by interacting with gut hormones and receptors.

Peptides such as motilin and glucagon-like peptide-1 (GLP-1) are key regulators of gut motility. Motilin stimulates the migrating motor complex (MMC). This pattern of contractions occurs between meals to clear the stomach and small intestine of residual food. GLP-1, on the other hand, slows gastric emptying, which ensures that nutrients are absorbed efficiently in the small intestine.

Peptides like vasoactive intestinal peptide (VIP) and substance P interact with receptors in the gut lining to modulate smooth muscle contractions. For instance, VIP promotes relaxation of the gut muscles, while substance P stimulates contractions. A 2019 review in Frontiers in Endocrinology emphasized the therapeutic potential of targeting these peptide-receptor interactions to treat motility disorders like IBS.

The gut-brain axis is a bidirectional communication system between the gut and the brain, and peptides play a key role in this connection. For example, ghrelin, a peptide produced in the stomach, stimulates appetite and influences gut motility, while GLP-1 regulates satiety and glucose metabolism. Disruptions in these peptides can result in conditions like obesity or eating disorders.

Peptides in Gut Lining Repair

The gut lining (intestinal epithelium) is a critical barrier that separates the gut's contents from the bloodstream. This single layer of cells absorbs nutrients while preventing harmful substances like bacteria, toxins, and undigested food particles from entering the bloodstream. When this barrier is compromised, it can cause chronic inflammation, autoimmune diseases, and a host of other health issues.

Enhancing Epithelial Cell Growth

The intestinal epithelium is a rapidly renewing tissue, with cells being replaced every three to five days. This constant turnover is necessary to maintain a healthy gut barrier. Peptides stimulate the growth and regeneration of epithelial cells, which ensures the gut lining remains intact and functional.

LL-37 and Defensins

These antimicrobial peptides (AMPs) protect against pathogens and promote epithelial cell proliferation. LL-37 is a cathelicidin-derived peptide that has been shown to enhance wound healing in the gut by stimulating the migration and growth of epithelial cells. A 2021 study published in Cellular and Molecular Gastroenterology and Hepatology demonstrated that LL-37 accelerates the repair of damaged intestinal epithelium, which makes it a potential therapeutic agent for conditions like IBD.

Growth Factors

Peptides such as transforming growth factor-beta (TGF-β) and epidermal growth factor (EGF) are also involved in epithelial cell regeneration. These peptides are naturally produced in the gut and maintain the integrity of the intestinal lining. For example, EGF has been shown to promote the healing of ulcers and other mucosal injuries in the gut.

Regulating Tight Junction Proteins

Tight junctions are protein complexes that act like sealants between intestinal epithelial cells, which prevent harmful substances from leaking into the bloodstream. When these junctions are disrupted, the gut becomes more permeable, which causes leaky gut syndrome. Peptides help maintain and restore tight junction integrity.

Zonulin-Modulating Peptides

Zonulin is a protein that regulates tight junctions. Elevated levels of zonulin are associated with increased intestinal permeability. Peptides that modulate zonulin activity, such as larazotide acetate, have been shown to restore tight junction function and reduce gut permeability. A 2020 study in Frontiers in Pharmacology highlighted the potential of larazotide acetate as a treatment for celiac disease and other conditions linked to leaky gut.

Collagen Peptides

Collagen is rich in amino acids like glycine and proline, which are necessary to synthesize tight junction proteins. Collagen peptides have been shown to strengthen the gut lining by promoting the production of these proteins. A 2019 study on nutrients found that collagen supplementation improved gut barrier function in patients with IBD.

Chronic inflammation is a major contributor to gut lining damage. Inflammatory conditions like IBD, Crohn's disease, and ulcerative colitis can weaken the intestinal barrier, which increases permeability. Peptides modulate immune responses and reduce inflammation, which protects the gut lining.

Cathelicidins

These antimicrobial peptides (e.g., LL-37) have potent anti-inflammatory properties. They inhibit the production of pro-inflammatory cytokines, such as TNF-α and IL-6, which are known to damage the gut lining. A 2022 review in Nature Reviews Gastroenterology & Hepatology emphasized the therapeutic potential of cathelicidins in treating inflammatory gut disorders.

Anti-inflammatory Peptides

Peptides like thymosin beta-4 and apelin have been shown to reduce inflammation and promote tissue repair in the gut. Thymosin beta-4, for example, reduces oxidative stress and inflammation, which accelerates the healing of mucosal injuries.

Supporting the Mucus Layer

The gut lining is covered by a mucus layer that acts as a protective shield, which traps harmful substances and prevents them from reaching the epithelial cells. Peptides maintain this mucus layer, which further supports gut barrier function.

Mucin-Stimulating Peptides

Mucins are glycoproteins that form the backbone of the mucus layer. Peptides like trefoil factor peptides (TFFs) stimulate the production of mucins, which ensures the mucus layer remains thick and functional.

Peptides and Microbiome Balance

The gut microbiome is a complex community of trillions of bacteria, viruses, fungi, and other microorganisms and is a cornerstone of human health. It plays a vital role in digestion, immunity, and even mental health through the gut-brain axis. When the balance of this microbiome is disrupted—a condition known as dysbiosis—it can result in a range of health issues, such as obesity, diabetes, IBD, and even mood disorders like anxiety and depression. The following are the mechanisms by which peptides support microbiome balance.

Antimicrobial Action

One of the most critical roles of peptides in the gut is their antimicrobial action. Certain peptides, particularly those produced by beneficial bacteria (probiotics), can selectively target harmful pathogens without disrupting the beneficial microbes. This targeted approach maintains a healthy microbiome.

- **Bacteriocins** are antimicrobial peptides produced by probiotic bacteria, such as Lactobacillus and Bifidobacterium. They disrupt the cell membranes of harmful bacteria and effectively neutralize them. For example, nisin, a well-studied bacteriocin, has been shown to inhibit the growth of pathogenic bacteria like Clostridium difficile and Staphylococcus aureus while sparing beneficial gut flora. A 2021 study in Frontiers in Microbiology highlighted the potential of bacteriocins as alternatives to antibiotics, which often disrupt the gut microbiome.
- **Defensins and Cathelicidins** are antimicrobial peptides produced by the gut's epithelial and immune cells. They defend against infections by targeting harmful bacteria, viruses, and fungi.

Immune Modulation

The gut is home to approximately seventy percent of the body's immune cells, which makes it a critical hub for immune function. Peptides modulate the immune response to microbial threats. This action ensures the immune system remains balanced and does not overreact to harmless or beneficial microbes.

- **Interaction with Immune Cells:** Peptides like LL-37 and thymosin alpha-1 interact with gut-associated immune cells, such as macrophages and dendritic cells, to regulate immune responses. For example, LL-37 has been shown to reduce the production of pro-inflammatory cytokines, such as TNF-α and IL-6, while promoting the release of anti-inflammatory cytokines like IL-10. This balanced immune response helps prevent chronic inflammation, which is often linked to dysbiosis and conditions like IBD.

- **Toll-Like Receptor (TLR) Modulation:** Peptides can also interact with Toll-like receptors (TLRs), which are proteins that recognize microbial patterns and trigger immune responses. By modulating TLR activity, peptides help ensure the immune system responds appropriately to microbial threats without excessive inflammation.

Prebiotic-Like Effects

In addition to their antimicrobial and immune-modulating effects, some peptides act as substrates for beneficial bacteria, which promote their growth and activity. These prebiotic-like effects help maintain a healthy and diverse microbiome.

- **Bioactive Peptides:** Certain peptides derived from dietary proteins, such as casein and whey, have been shown to promote the growth of beneficial bacteria like Lactobacillus and Bifidobacterium. These bacteria produce short-chain fatty acids (SCFAs), such as butyrate, which nourish the gut lining and regulate inflammation. Bioactive peptides from milk proteins enhance the growth of beneficial bacteria and improve gut health in individuals with IBS.

- **Collagen Peptides:** Collagen is rich in amino acids like glycine and proline, which serve as energy sources for beneficial bacteria. Collagen peptides have been shown to support the growth of Lactobacillus and Bifidobacterium while inhibiting pathogenic species like E. coli. A 2020 study in *Gut Microbes* highlighted the potential of collagen peptides as a dietary intervention to promote microbiome balance.

Supporting the Gut-Brain Axis

The gut microbiota is critical to the gut-brain axis, which is a bidirectional communication mechanism that connects the gut and the brain. Dysbiosis has been linked to mental health disorders like anxiety, depression, and even neurodegenerative diseases. Peptides contribute to this connection by supporting a healthy microbiome and reducing inflammation.

- **Neuroactive Peptides:** Peptides like ghrelin and GLP-1 not only regulate gut function but also influence brain activity. For example, GLP-1 has been shown to reduce inflammation in the gut and brain, which potentially improves symptoms of depression and anxiety. A 2021 study in Molecular Psychiatry highlighted the role of gut-derived peptides in mental health.

Peptides for Gut Disorders like IBD

IBD, such as Crohn's disease and ulcerative colitis, are chronic conditions characterized by inflammation of the gastrointestinal (GI) tract. These diseases can cause debilitating symptoms such as abdominal pain, diarrhea, weight loss, and fatigue, which can significantly impact a patient's quality of life. Although the exact cause of IBD remains unclear, it is believed to result from a combination of genetic, environmental, and immune factors, often accompanied by an imbalance in the gut microbiome.

Reducing Inflammation

Chronic inflammation is the hallmark of IBD, driven by an overactive immune response that damages the gut lining. Peptides help modulate this immune response, reduce inflammation, and alleviate symptoms.

- **LL-37:** This antimicrobial peptide is derived from cathelicidin and has potent anti-inflammatory properties. It inhibits the production of pro-inflammatory cytokines, such as TNF-α, IL-6, and IL-1β, which are elevated in IBD patients. LL-37 reduces inflammation and promotes tissue repair in animal models of colitis, which highlights its potential as a therapeutic agent for IBD.
- **Thymosin Beta-4**: This peptide is known for its anti-inflammatory and tissue-repairing properties. It reduces oxidative stress and promotes the healing of mucosal injuries in the gut. A 2020 review in Frontiers in Immunology highlighted the role of thymosin beta-4 in managing chronic inflammatory conditions, such as IBD.

Enhancing Mucosal Immunity

A mucus layer composed of mucins, which are glycoproteins that form a physical barrier against irritants and pathogens, protects the gut lining. In IBD, this mucus layer is often compromised, which leaves the gut lining vulnerable to damage. Peptides enhance mucosal immunity as they support the production of mucins and maintain the integrity of the mucus layer.

- **Trefoil Factor Peptides (TFFs):** These peptides maintain the mucus layer and promote mucosal healing. TFFs stimulate the production of mucins and enhance the migration of epithelial cells to repair damaged areas.
- **Mucin-Stimulating Peptides:** Certain peptides, such as those derived from dietary proteins, have been shown to enhance mucin production. For example, bioactive peptides from milk proteins (e.g., casein) have been found to support the mucus layer and protect the gut lining from irritants.

Restoring Gut Microbiota

Dysbiosis (an imbalance in the gut microbiome) is a key feature of IBD. Patients with IBD often have a reduced diversity of beneficial bacteria and an overgrowth of harmful pathogens. Peptides selectively target harmful bacteria and promote the growth of beneficial ones, which helps re-establish a healthy microbiome.

Supporting the Gut-Brain Axis

IBD is not just a physical condition; it also has significant psychological impacts. Many IBD patients experience anxiety, depression, and reduced quality of life. The gut-brain axis plays a key role in this connection. Peptides reduce inflammation and promote a healthy microbiome, which supports mental health.

Sources of Gut Health-Boosting Peptides

Fermented Foods

Fermented foods are rich in beneficial bacteria and the peptides they produce, which makes them a cornerstone of gut health. Examples include yogurt, kefir, miso, tempeh, sauerkraut, and kimchi.

Fermented foods contain probiotic-derived peptides, such as bacteriocins, which selectively target harmful bacteria and promote the growth of beneficial microbes. Fermented foods like kefir and kimchi enhance microbiome diversity and reduce inflammation thanks to their peptide content.

Bone Broth

Bone broth has gained popularity as a gut-healing food due to its high collagen content. Collagen peptides, such as glycine and proline, help repair the gut lining and maintain tight junction integrity. They improve gut barrier function and reduce inflammation in individuals with IBD.

Lean Proteins

Lean proteins, such as chicken, fish, eggs, and turkey, are excellent sources of bioactive peptides that support digestion and immune function. These proteins contain key peptides like lactoferrin and glutamine, which enhance nutrient absorption, reduce inflammation, and support immune responses. Bioactive peptides from chicken and fish also improve gut motility and reduce oxidative stress.

Plant-Based Sources

Plant-based foods are rich in peptides that act as substrates for beneficial bacteria that promote microbiome balance. Examples include Legumes (lentils, chickpeas), seeds (chia, flax), and whole grains (quinoa, oats).

These foods contain peptides with prebiotic-like effects, such as lunasin and defensins, which promote the growth of Lactobacillus and Bifidobacterium. Plant-based peptides enhance microbiome diversity and reduce inflammation in individuals with IBS.

Peptide Supplements

For patients who need additional support, peptide supplements can provide targeted benefits for gut health. The following are commonly used peptides.

- **Collagen Peptides:** Support gut lining repair and reduce inflammation.

- **Bovine Colostrum:** Rich in immunoglobulins and growth factors that enhance gut immunity and repair.
- **Antimicrobial Peptides (AMPs):** Target harmful bacteria and restore microbiome balance, e.g., nisin and LL-37.

Nursing Implications

Peptides provide a promising approach to help manage gut-related conditions, but their effectiveness depends on how well they are integrated into patient care plans. Below are practical nursing implications for using peptides to support gut health, tailored to help nurses educate, assess, and intervene effectively.

Educate Patients

- Explain the basics: Use simple language to explain what peptides are and how they help repair the gut lining, balance the microbiome, and reduce inflammation.
- Highlight food sources: Provide a list of peptide-rich foods and explain their benefits.
- Discuss supplements: If appropriate, educate patients about peptide supplements like collagen or bovine colostrum and emphasize their specific benefits.
- Address misconceptions: Peptides are not a "magic cure" but part of a holistic approach to gut health that includes diet, lifestyle, and medical treatment.

Identify Patients Who Can Benefit from Peptides

- Screen for gut health issues: Ask patients about symptoms such as bloating, diarrhea, constipation, abdominal pain, or food sensitivities, which may indicate gut dysfunction.
- Review medical history: Identify patients with conditions like IBS, IBD, leaky gut syndrome, or antibiotic-associated diarrhea, as they may benefit from peptide therapy.
- Assess dietary habits: Ask about the patient's diet to identify peptide intake gaps.
- Monitor for inflammation: Look for signs of chronic inflammation, such as fatigue, joint pain, or skin issues, which may be linked to gut health.

Incorporate Peptides into Patient Care

- Suggest peptide-rich foods like bone broth, fermented foods (yogurt, kefir, kimchi), lean proteins (chicken, fish, eggs), and plant-based sources (legumes, seeds).
- Provide simple recipes or meal ideas, such as adding bone broth to soups or using yogurt as a snack.
- Recommend high-quality peptide supplements, such as collagen peptides, bovine colostrum, or glutamine, based on the patient's needs.
- Advise on proper dosage and timing (e.g., collagen peptides in the morning or before meals).
- Encourage patients to pair peptide therapy with other gut-friendly practices. To boost gut health,

patients can reduce stress, stay hydrated, and avoid processed foods.

Monitor and Evaluate

- Track symptoms: Regularly ask patients about changes in their symptoms, such as reduced bloating, improved bowel movements, or increased energy levels.
- Monitor for side effects: Watch for potential side effects of peptide supplements, such as mild digestive discomfort, and adjust dosages accordingly.

Support Overall Well-Being

Gut health is deeply connected to overall health, including immunity, mental health, and chronic disease prevention. Nurses can advocate for a holistic approach that addresses all aspects of a patient's well-being.

Chapter 10: Peptides in Cancer Research and Treatment

Cancer remains one of the most challenging diseases to treat, with traditional therapies like chemotherapy and radiation often causing significant side effects due to their lack of specificity. In recent years, peptides have emerged as a promising tool in cancer research and treatment, as they provide a more targeted and less toxic approach. Peptides are short chains of amino acids that play diverse roles in biological processes, including cell signaling, immune modulation, and tissue repair. Their unique properties, such as high specificity, low toxicity, and ease of synthesis, make them ideal candidates for innovative cancer therapies.

Peptides in Cancer Therapy

Targeted Drug Delivery

One of the most significant advantages of peptides is their ability to deliver drugs directly to cancer cells, which minimizes damage to healthy tissues. This is achieved through peptide-drug conjugates (PDCs) that link a targeting peptide to a therapeutic agent. The peptide component binds to specific receptors overexpressed on cancer cells and delivers the drug directly to the tumor.

- Example: Lutetium-177-labeled peptides, such as Lutetium-177-DOTATATE, are used to treat neuroendocrine tumors. These peptides target somatostatin receptors on tumor cells and deliver radiation precisely to the cancer site.

Cytotoxic Peptides

Cytotoxic peptides are designed to induce apoptosis (programmed cell death) in cancer cells while sparing normal cells. These peptides disrupt cancer cell membranes or interfere with intracellular signaling pathways.

- Example: Bcl-2-inhibiting peptides block the activity of Bcl-2, a protein that prevents apoptosis in cancer cells. These peptides inhibit Bcl-2 and promote cancer cell death.

Angiogenesis Inhibition

Tumors require a blood supply to grow and metastasize. Peptides that inhibit angiogenesis (the formation of new blood vessels) can effectively starve tumors of nutrients. These peptides block pro-angiogenic factors like VEGF (vascular endothelial growth factor) or mimic anti-angiogenic proteins.

- Example: Thrombospondin-derived peptides mimic the anti-angiogenic effects of thrombospondin, a natural protein that inhibits blood vessel formation.

Peptides in Immune Modulation for Cancer Treatment

Cancer Vaccines

Cancer vaccines represent a groundbreaking advancement in oncology as they harness the body's immune system to fight cancer. Unlike regular vaccines that prevent infectious diseases, cancer vaccines are designed to activate the immune system to recognize and target existing tumor cells. Among the most promising types are peptide-based vaccines, which use tumor-specific peptides (neoantigens) to activate the immune system. Healthcare workers must understand the science behind these vaccines, their mechanisms of action, and their clinical applications to provide holistic, patient-centered care.

Peptide-based cancer vaccines are a form of immunotherapy that uses small fragments of proteins, called peptides, to stimulate an immune response against cancer cells. These peptides are derived from neoantigens, which are unique proteins produced by cancer cells due to mutations in their DNA. Because neoantigens are specific to cancer cells and not found in healthy tissues, they provide an ideal target for the immune system.

How Do Peptide-Based Cancer Vaccines Work?

- **Identify Neoantigens:** Each patient's tumor is analyzed through genomic sequencing to identify unique mutations that produce neoantigens. These neoantigens are then synthesized into peptides that can be used in the vaccine.
- **Activate T Cells:** The vaccine is usually administered to the patient via injection. The peptides are taken up by antigen-presenting cells (APCs), such as dendritic cells, which process and present the peptides on their surface. This presentation activates immune cells that can recognize and destroy cancer cells (i.e., T cells).
- **Target Cancer Cells:** Activated T cells seek out and destroy cancer cells that display the same

neoantigens throughout the body. This targeted approach minimizes damage to healthy tissues and reduces the risk of side effects.

Neoantigen-Based Personalized Cancer Vaccines

Personalized neoantigen vaccines are one of the most exciting developments in peptide-based cancer vaccines. These vaccines are tailored to each patient's unique tumor mutations, which makes them highly specific and effective.

- **Melanoma** is a type of skin cancer that has been a focus of neoantigen vaccine research due to its high mutation rate. In clinical trials, personalized neoantigen vaccines have successfully induced strong immune responses and improved survival rates.
- **Glioblastoma** is an aggressive brain cancer that has also been targeted with neoantigen vaccines. Early-phase clinical trials have shown that these vaccines can stimulate immune responses and extend progression-free survival in glioblastoma patients.

Advantages of Peptide-Based Cancer Vaccines

- **Specificity:** Because neoantigens are unique to cancer cells, peptide-based vaccines target tumors with high precision, sparing healthy tissues.
- **Personalization:** Each vaccine is tailored to the patient's unique tumor mutations, which increases the likelihood of success.

- **Reduced Toxicity:** Unlike chemotherapy and radiation, which can cause widespread damage, peptide-based vaccines are generally well-tolerated with minimal side effects.
- **Long-Lasting Immunity:** Peptide-based vaccines can induce memory T cells, which provide long-term protection against cancer recurrence.

Checkpoint Inhibitor Peptides

Immune checkpoint inhibitors are a breakthrough in cancer immunotherapy, and peptides are being developed to enhance their efficacy. These therapies target specific pathways that cancer cells use to evade the immune system, which allows the body's natural defenses to recognize and destroy tumors more effectively.

Mechanism: Peptides target immune checkpoint pathways like PD-1/PD-L1 and CTLA-4, which cancer cells exploit to evade immune detection. These pathways act as "brakes" on the immune system and prevent T cells from attacking cancer cells. Peptides block these checkpoints and restore the immune system's ability to recognize and destroy tumors.

- Example: PD-1/PD-L1 blocking peptides prevent cancer cells from deactivating T cells. When PD-1 on T cells binds to PD-L1 on cancer cells, it signals the T cell to stop attacking. Blocking this interaction allows T cells to remain active and continue targeting cancer cells. Drugs like pembrolizumab (Keytruda) and nivolumab (Opdivo) are examples of PD-1 inhibitors that have successfully treated cancers like melanoma, lung cancer, and renal cell carcinoma.

T-Cell Activation and Adoptive Immunotherapy

Peptides are also used to enhance T-cell responses in adoptive immunotherapy, where T cells are engineered to target cancer cells. This approach modifies a patient's own immune cells to improve their ability to recognize and destroy cancer cells, which provides a highly personalized and effective treatment option.

Mechanism: Peptides are used to modify T cells, which enables them to recognize and destroy cancer cells more effectively. In chimeric antigen receptor (CAR) therapy, T cells are extracted from the patient, genetically engineered to express a receptor that binds to a specific tumor antigen, and then infused back into the patient. These engineered T cells can then seek out and destroy cancer cells with precision.

- Example: Peptide-based CAR-T therapy engineers T cells to express receptors that bind to tumor-specific peptides. Therapies like tisagenlecleucel (Kymriah) and axicabtagene ciloleucel (Yescarta) target the CD19 protein on B-cells, which effectively treats B-cell malignancies like acute lymphoblastic leukemia (ALL) and non-Hodgkin lymphoma.

Peptides in Tumor Suppression and Metastasis Prevention

Cancer is not just a single disease but a complex process that involves uncontrolled cell growth, invasion, and metastasis. Even though traditional therapies like chemotherapy and radiation have been the mainstay of cancer treatment, they often come with significant side effects and limited efficacy in advanced stages. Peptides are uniquely able to target specific molecular pathways, which makes them powerful tools to suppress tumors and prevent metastasis.

Inhibition of Tumor Growth

Mechanism: Mutations in key genes that regulate cell proliferation and survival drive tumor growth. One of the most well-known oncogenic pathways involves the RAS family of proteins, which are mutated in approximately thirty percent of all human cancers, including pancreatic, colorectal, and lung cancers. RAS proteins become hyperactive when mutated and send constant signals for cells to grow and divide uncontrollably.

Peptides can be specifically designed to inhibit these oncogenic proteins. For example, RAS-inhibiting peptides bind to mutated RAS proteins, which block their ability to activate downstream signaling pathways that promote tumor growth.

- Example: In preclinical studies, KRAS(G12C) inhibitors have shown promise for targeting a specific mutation in the KRAS gene, which is common in lung and pancreatic cancers. The peptide blocks this mutation and effectively halts tumor proliferation.

Blocking Cancer Cell Migration and Invasion

Mechanism: Metastasis is the spread of cancer cells from the primary tumor to distant organs and is responsible for the majority of cancer-related deaths. For cancer cells to metastasize, they must detach from the primary tumor, invade surrounding tissues, enter the bloodstream, and establish new tumors in distant sites. Peptides target key molecules involved in cell migration and invasion, which disrupts this process.

Peptides can block integrins, which are proteins on the surface of cancer cells that help them attach to the extracellular matrix (ECM) and migrate through tissues. Peptides disrupt integrin function, which prevents cancer cells from spreading.

- Example: Integrin-blocking peptides (e.g., cilengitide) have been tested in clinical trials for their ability to inhibit metastasis in cancers like glioblastoma and melanoma. These peptides bind to integrins and prevent cancer cells from attaching to blood vessels and spreading to other parts of the body.

Peptides in Combination Therapy

Mechanism: Even though peptides alone can be effective, their true potential is often realized when combined with traditional therapies like chemotherapy, radiation, or immunotherapy. This approach is known as combination therapy and can enhance treatment efficacy, reduce the required dose of toxic drugs, and minimize side effects.

Peptides can sensitize cancer cells to other treatments by disrupting their survival mechanisms. For example, a peptide might block a protein that helps cancer cells repair DNA damage, which makes them more vulnerable to chemotherapy or radiation.

- Example: In breast and lung cancers, peptide-chemotherapy combinations have shown synergistic effects. A peptide called p28 has enhanced the effectiveness of chemotherapy drugs like doxorubicin by increasing their uptake into cancer cells.

Commonly Used Peptides in Tumor Suppression and Metastasis Prevention

The following are examples of peptides currently being used or studied in cancer therapy.

- **KRAS-inhibiting peptides** target mutations in the KRAS gene, which is common in lung and pancreatic cancers. A peptide-based drug called AMG 510 has shown promise in clinical trials for KRAS-mutated cancers.
- **Integrin-blocking peptides** prevent cancer cells from attaching to blood vessels and spreading. Cilengitide was tested in glioblastoma and melanoma.
- **p28 Peptide** enhances the effectiveness of chemotherapy by increasing drug uptake in cancer

cells. It is used in combination with doxorubicin for breast and lung cancers.

- **Tumor-penetrating peptides** help drugs penetrate deep into tumors, which improves their effectiveness. iRGD is a peptide that enhances drug delivery to tumors.

Challenges and Future Directions

Despite their promise, peptide-based therapies face several challenges, such as stability, bioavailability, and resistance mechanisms. Emerging research addresses these issues through the following mechanisms.

- **Peptide Nanotechnology:** Nanoparticles can improve peptide delivery and stability. They can protect peptides from degradation and enhance their uptake by cancer cells.
- **Synthetic Peptide Libraries:** High-throughput screening can identify novel peptides with therapeutic potential. These libraries allow researchers to rapidly test thousands of peptides for their ability to target specific cancer pathways.
- **Overcoming Resistance:** Researchers are creating peptides that target multiple pathways. Combination therapies that include these peptides can reduce the likelihood of resistance.

Nursing Implications

Patient Education

- Educate patients about the benefits and potential side effects of peptide-based therapies.

- Provide resources on peptide-rich diets and supplements that support overall health.

Monitoring and Assessment

- Regularly assess patients for side effects and treatment efficacy.
- Monitor for immune-related adverse events in patients receiving immunotherapy.

Supportive Care

- Provide symptom management for side effects like nausea, fatigue, and pain.
- Provide emotional support to patients undergoing cancer treatment.

Collaboration

- Advocate for personalized peptide-based therapies tailored to each patient's unique needs.

- Work closely with oncologists, dietitians, and other healthcare providers to develop comprehensive care plans.

Chapter 11: Peptides for Sleep and Stress Management

Mechanism of Peptides in Sleep and Stress Regulation

Peptides are critical modulators of neurotransmitter systems involved in sleep regulation and stress responses, with mechanisms supported by robust scientific evidence. Their interactions with key neural pathways provide insights into potential therapeutic applications.

Delta-Sleep-Inducing Peptide (DSIP) and GABAergic Modulation

DSIP enhances GABAergic activity, which is a primary inhibitory system in the CNS. It promotes GABA release and potentiates GABA-A receptor function. Studies demonstrate that DSIP administration increases slow-wave sleep (SWS) duration by twenty to thirty percent, which correlates with elevated GABA levels in the hypothalamus. DSIP may bind to thalamocortical neurons, which reduces glutamatergic excitability and fosters a transition to restorative sleep stages. Human trials note improved sleep maintenance in insomnia patients, with EEG patterns showing enhanced delta-wave activity. Furthermore, DSIP's anxiolytic effects are linked to its suppression of amygdala hyperactivity, which dampens stress-induced neural circuits.

Fish-Derived Peptides and HPA Axis Regulation

Bioactive peptides from salmon, tuna, and algae (valine-tyrosine-proline tripeptides) exhibit stress-resilient properties as they can modulate glucocorticoid receptor (GR) sensitivity and serotonin (5-HT) pathways. In rodent models, oral administration of these peptides reduced corticosterone levels by forty to fifty percent after chronic stress, which was comparable to SSRIs. Mechanistically, they upregulate hippocampal GR expression, which enhances negative feedback to the HPA axis, thereby curtailing corticotropin-releasing hormone (CRH) and ACTH overproduction. Concurrently, they boost prefrontal cortex serotonin synthesis via tryptophan hydroxylase activation, which mitigates anxiety-like behaviors. For example, tilapia-derived peptides lowered ACTH by thirty percent in stressed zebrafish with a parallel increase of 5-HT1A receptor binding.

HPA Axis Stabilization and Neurotransmitter Homeostasis

Chronic HPA axis activation depletes serotonin by upregulating monoamine oxidase (MAO) and disrupts dopamine circuits, which impairs reward processing and circadian rhythms. Peptides like DSIP and marine-derived analogs counteract this by normalizing cortisol rhythms, which preserves tryptophan availability for 5-HT synthesis. In stressed rats, peptide treatment restored hippocampal dopamine D1 receptor expression by twenty-five percent, which aligned with improved sleep-wake cycle regularity. This stabilization also mitigates glucocorticoid-induced oxidative damage in locus coeruleus noradrenergic neurons, which prevents hyperarousal states.

Clinical and Nursing Implications

Peptide-based nutraceuticals, such as lactium (derived from milk casein), show promise in human trials. They reduced subjective stress scores by thirty-five percent and improved sleep latency. DSIP analogs are in Phase II trials for insomnia, with preliminary data indicating a twenty percent increase in SWS without next-day sedation. Challenges include bioavailability, which prompted advances in nanoparticle delivery systems to enhance blood-brain barrier penetration.

When administering peptide-based therapies, nurses should monitor patients for changes in anxiety or sleep patterns. They must also understand neurotransmitter modulation to help educate patients about the biological basis of these treatments.

Modulation of Circadian Rhythms

Circadian rhythms are tightly linked to sleep quality and stress adaptation. Peptides such as CLIP/ACTH18-39 and DSIP influence circadian gene expression (e.g., Per2), which regulates sleep phases. Epitalon is a synthetic pineal peptide that extends lifespan and enhances melatonin secretion, which reinforces circadian alignment. Disrupted rhythms are common in shift workers and jet-lagged patients. They may benefit from peptide therapies that reset biological clocks.

Nursing Implication: Patients should be educated on maintaining consistent sleep schedules alongside peptide use. For shift workers, consider timed administration of circadian-modulating peptides like Epitalon.

Popular Peptides for Sleep & Stress Management

DSIP

DSIP is a nonapeptide that reduces ACTH and corticosterone levels, which mitigates stress-induced sleep fragmentation. In mice, DSIP administration increased lifespan and reduced tumor incidence, which suggests systemic benefits. Its ability to stabilize GABA and serotonin pathways makes it a treatment candidate for insomnia and anxiety disorders.

Nursing Implication: Patients using DSIP must be monitored for sedation or hypotension. Due to altered metabolism, dose adjustments may be needed for older adult patients.

Selank

Selank (Thr-Lys-Pro-Arg-Pro-Gly-Pro) is a synthetic heptapeptide derived from tuftsin. It demonstrates anxiolytic effects by modulating serotonin (5-HT) and GABA systems, which is distinct from traditional sedative anxiolytics. Preclinical studies reveal its dual action.

- **Serotonergic Enhancement:** Selank inhibits serotonin reuptake and upregulates tryptophan hydroxylase (TPH2) activity, which increases extracellular serotonin in the prefrontal cortex. Selank elevated hippocampal 5-HT levels in stressed rats by forty percent compared to controls.

This result is akin to low-dose SSRIs but without sexual side effects.

- **GABAergic Modulation:** Selank activates the amygdala's glutamic acid decarboxylase (GAD65/67), which boosts GABA synthesis. A 2017 Psychopharmacology study showed that it reduced GABA transaminase activity by twenty-five percent, which prolonged GABA's inhibitory effects. As Selank does not bind to GABA-A receptors, patients can avoid sedation and dependence, unlike benzodiazepines.
- **Stress Resilience and Comparative Mechanisms:** Selank shares functional overlap with DSIP and CLIP in stress-axis regulation. Like DSIP, Selank attenuates HPA axis hyperactivity. Intranasal Selank (0.15 mg/kg) reduced cortisol by twenty-two percent during acute stress tests in humans. Similar to CLIP, Selank promotes post-stress recovery. In sleep-deprived mice, REM sleep increased by thirty percent during recovery phases, which is linked to normalized CRH in the hypothalamus.

Nursing Implications

Drug Interactions

- SSRIs (e.g., sertraline): The risk of serotonin syndrome is low but possible; monitor for tremors and hyperreflexia.
- Benzodiazepines: Synergistic GABA effects may cause over-sedation. Avoid concurrent use in older adult patients.

Patient Education

- Delayed Onset: The effects manifest over seven to ten days due to neuroadaptive changes (e.g., dendritic remodeling in the amygdala). Advise against abrupt discontinuation.
- Administration: Teach proper intranasal technique (e.g., alternating nostrils) to optimize bioavailability (forty to fifty percent vs. ten percent oral).
- Monitoring: Assess for rare side effects, such as mild dizziness (eight percent of users) or nasal irritation (twelve percent).
- Screen for a history of autoimmune disorders: Selank may modulate IL-6, which poses theoretical risks in rheumatoid arthritis.

Contraindications

- Pregnancy: No human data; animal studies show embryotoxicity at high doses.

Epitalon (Epithalamin)

Epitalon is derived from pineal gland extracts. It regulates melatonin and extends telomeres, which delay aging-related sleep disturbances. It also enhances REM sleep and reduces oxidative stress, which supports long-term resilience.

Nursing Implication: This medication is ideal for older adult patients with age-related insomnia. To maximize its efficacy, monitor for melatonin sensitivity and adjust light exposure.

Oxytocin

Oxytocin is a neuropeptide produced in the hypothalamus. It dampens cortisol secretion and fosters social bonding, which reduces stress and modulates sleep.

In stressed individuals, intranasal oxytocin administration has been shown to reduce cortisol levels by up to twenty-six percent during social conflict tasks. This cortisol-lowering effect is linked to oxytocin's inhibition of amygdala hyperactivity, which is the fear-processing region of the brain. This, in turn, reduces downstream activation of the HPA axis. Beyond stress, oxytocin's influence extends to sleep architecture, particularly in populations with trauma-related disorders. For example, a 2016 trial involving PTSD patients revealed that nightly intranasal oxytocin (40 IU) over six weeks stabilized REM sleep patterns, which reduced nighttime awakenings by thirty-five percent and improved self-reported sleep quality.

These effects are attributed to oxytocin's ability to enhance functional connectivity between the prefrontal cortex and limbic regions, which regulates emotional memory processing during REM cycles.

However, oxytocin's vasodilatory properties necessitate cautious use in patients with cardiovascular conditions. Rodent studies have shown that high-dose oxytocin can transiently lower blood pressure by 10–15 mmHg and increase heart rate variability. This effect poses risks for individuals with preexisting hypotension or arrhythmias.

In clinical practice, nurses should screen for cardiovascular history and monitor vital signs during initial dosing. Patient education is equally critical as improper nasal administration, such as tilting the head back or rapid inhalation, can divert the peptide to the gastrointestinal tract. This reduces bioavailability by up to seventy percent. Training patients to administer doses in a seated position with a slow, steady breath optimizes absorption through the nasal mucosa. Additionally, patients should be advised that therapeutic benefits, such as reduced anxiety or improved sleep, may take weeks to manifest and require adherence to dosing schedules.

Although generally well-tolerated, nasal irritation occurs in twenty percent of users, which necessitates symptom monitoring and reassurance about its transient nature.

CRF Antagonists

CRF antagonists block stress-induced REM suppression. They also inhibit CRH receptors, which prevents HPA overactivation. This action makes them useful for chronic stress and depression.

Nursing Implication: Watch for adrenal insufficiency symptoms (e.g., hypotension). Pair with psychotherapy for comprehensive stress management.

Role of Peptides in Hormonal Balance for Sleep and Stress

Growth hormone-releasing peptides (GHRPs), such as GHRP-6 and hexarelin, stimulate ghrelin receptors in the hypothalamus, which enhances SWS, the deepest and most restorative phase of sleep. This activation triggers a cascade that amplifies growth hormone (GH) secretion, which is intrinsically tied to SWS regulation. In a pivotal human study, intravenous administration of GHRP-6 increased SWS duration by approximately thirty percent in healthy young adults. This result correlates with elevated GH levels measured during the first half of the night. This aligns with the natural circadian rhythm of GH, which peaks during early sleep, particularly in sync with SWS. For patients with GH deficiency conditions linked to fragmented sleep and reduced SWS, GHRPs restore GH secretion and improve sleep quality, as shown in clinical trials where nightly use of hexarelin improved subjective sleep scores and daytime fatigue in adults with pituitary dysfunction.

However, the metabolic effects of GH necessitate careful clinical management. GH antagonizes insulin signaling in skeletal muscle and liver, which induces transient insulin resistance. This mechanism was observed in studies where GH replacement therapy increased fasting glucose levels by ten to fifteen percent in deficient patients. Similarly, GHRP use may exacerbate hyperglycemia, particularly in individuals with preexisting insulin resistance. For example, a trial in older adults using GHRP-2 reported a twenty percent rise in postprandial glucose levels, which underscored the need for vigilant glucose monitoring. Nursing protocols emphasize bedtime administration of GHRPs to synchronize with endogenous GH pulses, which maximizes therapeutic efficacy and minimizes circadian disruption. Additionally, clinicians are advised to screen for diabetes risk factors and implement routine glucose checks, especially during initial treatment phases, to mitigate metabolic complications. This dual aim to optimize sleep recovery and manage metabolic side effects highlights the nuanced role of GHRPs in balancing hormonal health and patient safety.

Cortisol Reduction and Stress Control

Peptides like fish hydrolysate and DSIP lower cortisol, which prevents chronic stress damage. This is vital for patients with Cushing's syndrome or burnout.

Nursing Implication: Regularly assess adrenal function and electrolyte balance during peptide therapy to avoid hypocortisolism.

Effects of Peptides on Sleep Quality and Stress Resilience

Enhancement of Sleep Architecture

DSIP and CLIP prolong REM sleep, which is essential for emotional processing. Fish peptides increase SWS, aiding physical restoration.

Reduction of Anxiety and Improvement in Mood

Prolactin is induced by stress and enhances REM rebound and serotonin synthesis. Peptides like Selank amplify this effect, which reduces anxiety without cognitive impairment.

Influence on Relaxation and Recovery

Peptides accelerate post-stress recovery by lowering oxidative stress and inflammation. Fish hydrolysate, for example, improves mitochondrial function, which aids in cellular repair.

Chapter 12: 150 Peptides (Dosage guide)

Muscle Growth & Fat Loss Peptide Protocols

CJC-1295 with DAC + Ipamorelin – CJC-1295 with DAC 2 mg once weekly + Ipamorelin 300 mcg daily. Stimulates growth hormone release to support lean muscle growth, fat reduction, and improved recovery.

MK-677 (Ibutamoren) – 10–25 mg orally daily. Stimulates natural GH and IGF-1 release to promote muscle gain, fat loss, better sleep, and recovery.

Tesamorelin – 2 mg subcutaneously daily. FDA-approved to reduce visceral adipose tissue. Used off-label for body re-composition and fat loss.

AOD-9604 – 300–500 mcg subcutaneously once daily, preferably in the morning. Mimics the fat-burning activity of HGH without affecting blood sugar or growth.

HGH Fragment 176-191 – 250–500 mcg subcutaneously 1–2x daily, ideally in a fasted state in the morning or pre-workout. Targets fat loss through enhanced lipolysis without full GH effects.

IGF-1 LR3 – 20–50 mcg subcutaneously post-workout, up to 5 days per week. Boosts muscle cell proliferation and recovery, and promotes fat oxidation.

PEG-MGF (Mechano Growth Factor) – 200–400 mcg subcutaneously 2–3x per week. Supports muscle repair, hypertrophy, and satellite cell activation after workouts.

BPC-157 + TB-500 – BPC-157 250 mcg daily + TB-500 2–5 mg weekly. Enhances muscle and soft tissue healing, reduces inflammation, and accelerates recovery.

GHRP-6 + Mod GRF 1-29 – GHRP-6 100 mcg + Mod GRF 1-29 100 mcg 2–3x daily. Stimulates GH release, increases appetite, supports muscle building and fat metabolism.

Hexarelin – 100 mcg subcutaneously 1–2x daily. Potent GH secretagogue that promotes muscle hypertrophy and fat breakdown.

Follistatin 344 – 100–300 mcg intramuscularly weekly for short cycles. Inhibits myostatin to significantly increase muscle mass and strength.

5-Amino-1MQ – 50–100 mg orally daily. Modulates NNMT activity to boost metabolism and enhance fat loss during cutting or re-composition phases.

MOTS-c – 10–15 mg subcutaneously 2–3x weekly. Improves mitochondrial function, insulin sensitivity, and metabolic efficiency to aid fat loss and endurance.

Tesofensine – 0.25–0.5 mg orally daily. Powerful appetite suppressant with stimulant effects, used for rapid fat loss and metabolic enhancement.

Epitalon + CJC-1295 (no DAC) – Epitalon 10 mg daily for 10–20 days + CJC-1295 (no DAC) 100 mcg 1–2x daily.

Anti-aging and fat-loss combined to support sleep, metabolism, and GH release.

Cognitive Enhancement Peptide Protocols

Semax (N-Acetyl variant) – 300–600 mcg intranasally 1–2x daily. Enhances BDNF expression, and improves memory, focus, and stress resilience.

Selank – 250–500 mcg intranasally 1–2x daily. Anxiolytic and nootropic effects to support mood balance, mental clarity, and learning under stress.

Dihexa – 8–20 mg orally or transdermally daily. Powerful neurogenic peptide that may promote synaptogenesis and cognitive regeneration.

Cerebrolysin – 1–5 mL intramuscularly or intravenously daily for short cycles of 10–20 days. Supports neurorepair, memory, and recovery post brain injury or fatigue.

P21 Peptide – 500 mcg subcutaneously daily or EOD in short cycles of 2–4 weeks. Neuroprotective that enhances working memory and neuron regeneration (research compound).

NRG-1 (Neuregulin-1) – 50–100 mcg subcutaneously 2–3x weekly. Improves neural plasticity and learning. Also being explored for Alzheimer's and cognitive recovery.

NA-1 (Tat-NR2B9c) – 1–2 mg subcutaneously post-ischemic events or in neuroprotection cycles. Inhibits excitotoxicity and studied for stroke-related cognitive protection.

RG3 (Ginsenoside-RG3 peptide blend) – 100–200 mcg subcutaneously daily. May modulate dopamine and acetylcholine pathways to enhance clarity and alertness.

GHK-Cu – 2–3 mg subcutaneously or transdermally daily. Improves neurogenesis, wound healing, and cognitive aging through anti-inflammatory and regenerative effects.

BDNF Mimetics (experimental) – Dose based on analog type, such as 1–2 mg subcutaneously. Supports neurogenesis and is being studied in age-related cognitive decline.

N-Acetyl Selank + Semax Stack – Selank 300 mcg + Semax 400 mcg intranasally 1–2x daily. Synergistic effect for focus, stress resilience, and memory consolidation.

Epitalon – 10 mg daily for 10–20 days per quarter. Supports pineal function, sleep cycle regulation, and neuroendocrine balance that impacts cognitive health.

DSIP (Delta Sleep-Inducing Peptide) – 100–200 mcg subcutaneously before bed. Improves sleep architecture which indirectly enhances memory consolidation and learning.

Thymosin Alpha-1 – 1.5 mg subcutaneously 2x per week. Immune-enhancing peptide that may improve cognition in cases of inflammation-driven brain fog or stress.

Lion's Mane Peptide Extract (experimental) – 1–2 mg orally or subcutaneously daily. Mimics the neurotrophic effects of Hericium erinaceus and supports NGF production and brain plasticity.

Anti-Aging & Longevity

Epitalon – 10 mg daily for 10–20 days per quarter. Promotes telomere elongation, improves pineal function and sleep regulation, and may increase lifespan markers.

Thymalin – 10–20 mg intramuscularly daily for 5–10 days. Immunomodulating peptide that supports thymus rejuvenation and immune system balance.

Thymosin Beta-4 (TB-500) – 2–5 mg subcutaneously once weekly. Enhances tissue repair, reduces systemic inflammation, and may support cellular regeneration.

GHK-Cu – 2–3 mg subcutaneously or transdermally daily. Copper-binding peptide that improves skin elasticity, wound healing, hair growth, and DNA repair signaling.

Foxo4-DRI – 5–10 mg subcutaneously 1–2x weekly for research use. Selectively removes senescent cells. Also being studied for rejuvenation and age-related disease mitigation.

Humanin (HNG) – 1–10 mg subcutaneously 2–3x weekly. Mitochondrial-derived peptide that protects neurons, cardiovascular tissue, and metabolic balance.

MOTS-c – 10–15 mg subcutaneously 2–3x per week. Improves mitochondrial efficiency, insulin sensitivity, and metabolic health in aging individuals.

CJC-1295 with DAC + Ipamorelin – CJC-1295 with DAC 2 mg weekly + Ipamorelin 300 mcg daily. Supports youthful GH secretion to enhance recovery, metabolism, and lean tissue.

KPV Peptide – 500 mcg subcutaneously daily or orally. Anti-inflammatory tripeptide that helps combat chronic low-grade inflammation or inflammaging.

BPC-157 – 250 mcg subcutaneously daily or orally. Supports tissue regeneration and gut health and protects against oxidative stress-related degeneration.

Tesamorelin – 2 mg subcutaneously daily. Shown to reduce visceral fat and improve metabolic profiles. It is particularly useful in aging populations.

IGF-1 LR3 – 20–50 mcg post-workout, max 5 days per week. Supports muscle maintenance and neuro-regeneration. It is useful in sarcopenia prevention.

NAD+ or NAD+ Precursors (such as NMN/Nicotinamide Riboside) – 100–500 mg orally daily or NAD+ 250 mg IV weekly. Supports mitochondrial health, energy metabolism, and cellular repair.

DSIP (Delta Sleep-Inducing Peptide) – 100–200 mcg before bed. Improves sleep quality and indirectly supports cognitive longevity and hormonal balance.

Melanotan II (low dose) – 250 mcg subcutaneously every 2–3 days. Stimulates melanin production for UV protection. It may also enhance libido and mood in aging individuals.

Healing & Recovery

BPC-157 – 250–500 mcg subcutaneously near the injury site or orally daily. Accelerates healing of muscles, tendons, ligaments, nerves, and gut lining.

TB-500 (Thymosin Beta-4) – 2–5 mg subcutaneously once or twice weekly. Promotes angiogenesis and cellular regeneration and is widely used for soft tissue and joint repair.

GHK-Cu – 2–3 mg subcutaneously or transdermally daily. Supports skin, hair, and connective tissue repair, with strong anti-inflammatory and regenerative properties.

CJC-1295 with DAC + Ipamorelin – CJC-1295 with DAC 2 mg once weekly + Ipamorelin 300 mcg daily. Enhances recovery through increased growth hormone and IGF-1 release.

Pentadecapeptide BPC-157 + TB-500 Stack – BPC-157 250 mcg + TB-500 2 mg subcutaneously daily. Powerful combination for joint, tendon, and muscle regeneration.

KPV Peptide – 200–500 mcg subcutaneously or orally daily. Potent anti-inflammatory that accelerates healing of internal organs, skin, and gut lining.

AOD-9604 – 300 mcg subcutaneously daily. Assists in fat-related injury repair and supports joint health due to regenerative effects on cartilage and soft tissues.

Epitalon – 10 mg daily for 10–20 days per quarter. Enhances cellular repair and regeneration. It is used in post-surgical and chronic healing applications.

IGF-1 LR3 – 20–40 mcg subcutaneously post-exercise, up to 5 days per week. Promotes muscle cell repair and regeneration following injury or intense training.

CGRP Fragment (experimental) – 50–100 mcg subcutaneously as needed. Enhances wound healing and angiogenesis. It is being studied for trauma and ischemic injury.

Semax – 300 mcg intranasally 1–2x daily. Supports neuro-regeneration and post-traumatic brain recovery. It also aids in stress-related recovery.

Selank – 250–500 mcg intranasally 1–2x daily. Improves recovery in anxiety-driven healing delays and supports immune stabilization.

Humanin (HNG) – 1–10 mg subcutaneously 2–3x weekly. Supports mitochondrial recovery and protects tissues from oxidative and inflammatory damage.

LL-37 – 100–200 mcg subcutaneously daily. Antimicrobial peptides are used to aid in chronic wound healing and reduce infection-related healing delays.

Thymosin Alpha-1 – 1.5 mg subcutaneously 2x per week. Modulates immune response and accelerates healing in individuals with chronic inflammation or infection.

Cardiovascular & Metabolic

MOTS-c – 10–15 mg subcutaneously 2–3x per week. Improves insulin sensitivity, supports mitochondrial health, and regulates fat and glucose metabolism.

5-Amino-1MQ – 50–100 mg orally daily. Reduces NNMT activity to boost NAD+ availability and enhance metabolic rate, fat loss, and blood glucose control.

Tesamorelin – 2 mg subcutaneously daily. FDA-approved to reduce visceral adiposity, particularly in metabolic syndrome and lipodystrophy cases.

Thymosin Beta-4 (TB-500) – 2–5 mg subcutaneously weekly. Promotes cardiac muscle regeneration, vascular repair, and anti-fibrotic activity post cardiac injury.

Epitalon – 10 mg subcutaneously daily for 10–20 days per quarter. Improves cardiovascular function through melatonin modulation and telomere restoration.

CJC-1295 with DAC + Ipamorelin – CJC-1295 with DAC 2 mg weekly + Ipamorelin 300 mcg daily. Enhances GH/IGF-1 axis and indirectly improves lipid metabolism and vascular tone.

GLP-1 Analogs (such as Semaglutide) – 0.25–1.0 mg subcutaneously weekly. Enhances insulin secretion, reduces appetite, supports weight loss, and protects cardiovascular tissue.

GHK-Cu – 2–3 mg subcutaneously or transdermally daily. Promotes vascular remodeling, improves endothelial function, and reduces oxidative stress.

Humanin (HNG) – 1–10 mg subcutaneously 2–3x weekly. Protects against atherosclerosis and insulin resistance through mitochondrial stress modulation.

Melanotan II (low dose) – 250 mcg subcutaneously every 2–3 days. Improves energy balance, increases lipolysis, and has potential cardiovascular protective effects.

KPV Peptide – 200–500 mcg subcutaneously or orally daily. Anti-inflammatory action reduces metabolic syndrome risk driven by chronic inflammation.

IGF-1 LR3 – 20–40 mcg subcutaneously post-workout, up to 5 days per week. Improves lean mass and insulin sensitivity, especially in age-related metabolic decline.

BPC-157 – 250 mcg subcutaneously daily or orally. Promotes healing of endothelial tissue and protects against cardiovascular stress and GI vascular damage.

DSIP (Delta Sleep-Inducing Peptide) – 100–200 mcg subcutaneously before bed. Supports blood pressure normalization through improved sleep and HPA axis regulation.

LL-37 – 100–200 mcg subcutaneously daily. Antimicrobial and immune-modulating peptide that may reduce systemic inflammation which contributes to vascular damage.

Mood & Stress

Selank – 250–500 mcg intranasally 1–2x daily. Anxiolytic peptide that modulates GABA and serotonin systems to reduce anxiety and enhance emotional stability.

Semax (N-Acetyl variant) – 300–600 mcg intranasally 1–2x daily. Supports mood regulation, improves focus, and reduces stress-induced cognitive decline.

DSIP (Delta Sleep-Inducing Peptide) – 100–200 mcg subcutaneously before bed. Promotes deep restorative sleep and regulates cortisol secretion under stress.

Oxytocin (Peptide) – 10–24 IU intranasally as needed. Social bonding peptide that improves mood and trust and reduces symptoms of social anxiety and depression.

Thymosin Alpha-1 – 1.5 mg subcutaneously 2x per week. Modulates immune-brain interaction and is shown to improve mood and resilience in chronic stress and fatigue.

CJC-1295 with DAC + Ipamorelin – CJC-1295 with DAC 2 mg weekly + Ipamorelin 300 mcg daily. Supports GH release and indirectly stabilizes mood and sleep-wake cycles.

Humanin (HNG) – 1–10 mg subcutaneously 2–3x per week. Mitochondrial peptide that enhances mood by protecting against oxidative and metabolic brain stress.

Epitalon – 10 mg subcutaneously daily for 10–20 days per quarter. Improves sleep and pineal function. Helps regulate circadian rhythm and emotional well-being.

BDNF Mimetics (experimental) – 1–2 mg subcutaneously 3x per week. Supports neuroplasticity and has antidepressant-like effects through BDNF pathway enhancement.

GHK-Cu – 2–3 mg subcutaneously or transdermally daily. Reduces oxidative stress and inflammation to improve mood and brain aging.

KPV Peptide – 200–500 mcg subcutaneously or orally daily. Reduces systemic inflammation, which contributes to stress-induced mood disorders.

Melanotan II (low dose) – 250 mcg subcutaneously every 2–3 days. May enhance mood, libido, and emotional resilience in some users.

N-Acetyl Selank + Semax Stack – Selank 300 mcg + Semax 400 mcg intranasally 1–2x daily. Synergistic mood and cognition enhancement combined with anti-anxiety benefits.

Thymalin – 10–20 mg intramuscularly daily for 5–10 days. Supports neuroendocrine balance and may improve mental clarity and resilience in stress.

BPC-157 – 250 mcg subcutaneously or orally daily. Gut-brain axis modulator that may improve stress response by reducing systemic and neural inflammation.

Sleep

DSIP (Delta Sleep-Inducing Peptide) – 100–200 mcg subcutaneously 30–60 minutes before bed. Promotes deep, restorative sleep by modulating sleep-wake cycles and reducing cortisol.

Epitalon – 10 mg subcutaneously daily for 10–20 days, quarterly. Enhances melatonin production and circadian rhythm alignment for improved sleep quality.

Selank – 250–500 mcg intranasally in the evening. Reduces anxiety and mental hyperactivity to support a smoother transition into sleep.

Semax – 300–600 mcg intranasally in the morning or midday. Improves cognitive fatigue during the day and indirectly supports better nighttime sleep.

CJC-1295 with DAC + Ipamorelin – CJC-1295 with DAC 2 mg weekly + Ipamorelin 300 mcg daily before bed. Enhances natural GH pulse during sleep for recovery and deeper rest.

Oxytocin (Peptide) – 10–24 IU intranasally 30–60 minutes before bed. Calms the nervous system and improves sleep onset through anxiolytic action.

Thymosin Alpha-1 – 1.5 mg subcutaneously 2x per week, evening preferred. Modulates immune-neuro interactions and may improve sleep during illness or stress.

BPC-157 – 250 mcg subcutaneously or orally at night. Reduces systemic inflammation and promotes gut-brain relaxation to aid in sleep onset.

GHK-Cu – 2–3 mg subcutaneously or transdermally in the evening. May improve sleep by reducing oxidative stress and restoring circadian balance.

KPV Peptide – 200–500 mcg subcutaneously or orally at night. Anti-inflammatory peptide that supports rest by calming peripheral and central nervous inflammation.

Melanotan II (low dose) – 250 mcg subcutaneously in the evening, 2–3x per week. Indirectly improves sleep through mood enhancement and light sensitivity modulation.

IGF-1 LR3 – 20–40 mcg post-evening workout, max 5x per week. Promotes deep recovery phases of sleep when dosed earlier in the evening.

MOTS-c – 10–15 mg subcutaneously in the morning, 2–3x per week. Regulates mitochondrial circadian signals which enhance nighttime recovery and metabolic resetting.

Thymalin – 10–20 mg intramuscularly daily for 5–10 days. Supports neuroendocrine balance and improved pineal gland signaling for restful sleep.

N-Acetyl Selank + DSIP Stack – Selank 300 mcg intranasal + DSIP 200 mcg subcutaneously before bed. Powerful calming and sleep-inducing combination that reduces anxiety and promotes deep sleep architecture.

Immune Modulation

Thymosin Alpha-1 (Tα1) – 1.5 mg subcutaneously 2x per week. Boosts T-cell function, regulates cytokine production, and enhances resistance to infections and immune dysregulation.

Thymalin – 10–20 mg intramuscularly daily for 5–10 days. Rejuvenates the thymus gland, modulates immune homeostasis, and restores immune competence in aging or illness.

BPC-157 – 250 mcg subcutaneously or orally daily. Promotes gut-immune balance, reduces systemic inflammation, and supports healing of mucosal immune barriers.

LL-37 – 100–200 mcg subcutaneously daily in short cycles. Antimicrobial peptide that enhances innate immunity and helps combat viral, bacterial, and fungal pathogens.

KPV Peptide – 200–500 mcg subcutaneously or orally daily. Tripeptide with strong anti-inflammatory and immunoregulatory effects, especially for gut and skin immune responses.

GHK-Cu – 2–3 mg subcutaneously or transdermally daily. Supports tissue repair and balances immune activity through anti-inflammatory and antioxidant pathways.

Epitalon – 10 mg subcutaneously daily for 10–20 days, quarterly. Enhances melatonin production and immune-endocrine regulation for longevity and defense.

VIP (Vasoactive Intestinal Peptide) – 100–200 mcg subcutaneously daily. Regulates Th1/Th2 balance. It is used in chronic inflammatory or autoimmune conditions like CIRS.

CJC-1295 with DAC + Ipamorelin – CJC-1295 with DAC 2 mg weekly + Ipamorelin 300 mcg daily. Boosts immune resilience through improved sleep, recovery, and hormonal restoration.

Humanin (HNG) – 1–10 mg subcutaneously 2–3x per week. Mitochondrial peptide that reduces inflammation and supports immune protection in aging or stress.

MOTS-c – 10–15 mg subcutaneously 2–3x per week. Enhances cellular stress response and immunity through mitochondrial signaling.

IGF-1 LR3 – 20–40 mcg post-exercise, max 5x per week. Supports immune regeneration and tissue healing following physical or oxidative stress.

Selank – 250–500 mcg intranasally 1–2x per day. Immunomodulatory and anti-inflammatory properties. It is useful in immune-sensitive anxiety or post-viral fatigue.

Semax – 300–600 mcg intranasally 1–2x per day. Indirectly modulates immune-neuro balance and supports mental clarity and recovery during immune stress.

Thymosin Beta-4 (TB-500) – 2–5 mg subcutaneously weekly. Supports immune cell migration and wound healing and suppresses chronic inflammatory cascades.

Sexual Function

T-141 (Bremelanotide) – 1–2 mg subcutaneously 30–60 minutes before sexual activity. FDA-approved to enhance libido and arousal in both men and women without affecting vascular function.

Melanotan II (low dose) – 250–500 mcg subcutaneously 2–3x per week. Increases sexual desire, spontaneous erections, and sensitivity through melanocortin receptor activation.

Oxytocin (Peptide) – 10–24 IU intranasally as needed. Promotes emotional bonding, increases trust, and enhances orgasm intensity and sexual satisfaction.

Kisspeptin-10 – 100 mcg subcutaneously 3x per week. Stimulates GnRH release to support testosterone and LH levels for improved libido and fertility.

Gonadorelin (GnRH) – 100–200 mcg subcutaneously 1–2x daily, pulsed. Boosts endogenous LH/FSH to support testosterone production and reproductive function.

CJC-1295 with DAC + Ipamorelin – CJC-1295 with DAC 2 mg weekly + Ipamorelin 300 mcg daily. Supports GH/IGF-1 levels to improve sexual energy, endurance, and hormonal balance.

BPC-157 – 250 mcg subcutaneously or orally daily. Promotes penile tissue healing and nitric oxide function. It is useful in erectile dysfunction caused by injury or inflammation.

Thymosin Beta-4 (TB-500) – 2–5 mg subcutaneously weekly. Supports vascular repair and smooth muscle regeneration in sexual tissues to enhance function over time.

GHK-Cu – 2–3 mg subcutaneously or transdermally daily. Improves blood flow and tissue regeneration in sexual organs, especially in aging populations.

Epitalon – 10 mg subcutaneously daily for 10–20 days, quarterly. Enhances pineal function and circadian rhythm. Improves testosterone regulation and sexual health.

MOTS-c – 10–15 mg subcutaneously 2–3x per week. Boosts mitochondrial energy and physical performance to support libido and stamina.

Tesamorelin – 2 mg subcutaneously daily. Supports GH axis and reduces visceral fat to improve hormonal profiles and sexual health in men.

IGF-1 LR3 – 20–40 mcg subcutaneously post-workout, max 5x per week. Enhances sexual recovery, erectile tissue repair, and anabolic drive.

LL-37 – 100–200 mcg subcutaneously daily. Indirectly supports sexual health by reducing chronic infections such as prostatitis or urogenital inflammation.

Selank – 250–500 mcg intranasally 1–2x daily. Reduces anxiety and emotional stress to improve libido and sexual performance in stress-related dysfunction.

Skin & Hair

GHK-Cu – 2–3 mg subcutaneously or transdermally daily. Stimulates collagen and elastin production. Improves wound healing, reduces fine lines, and promotes hair follicle health.

BPC-157 – 250 mcg subcutaneously near the affected area or orally daily. Accelerates healing of skin injuries and scars and supports GI-skin axis health.

Epitalon – 10 mg subcutaneously daily for 10–20 days per quarter. Improves skin elasticity and regeneration through telomerase activation and circadian rhythm regulation.

Thymosin Beta-4 (TB-500) – 2–5 mg subcutaneously weekly. Supports wound healing, reduces inflammation, and promotes angiogenesis in damaged or aging skin.

Melanotan II (low dose) – 250 mcg subcutaneously every 2–3 days. Stimulates melanin production and offers natural tanning and UV protection, with potential anti-aging benefits for skin.

IGF-1 LR3 – 20–40 mcg subcutaneously post-exercise or locally to scalp 3–5x per week. Promotes hair follicle cycling and regeneration, especially in thinning hair.

Copper Tripeptide-1 (GHK-Cu Topical) – apply topically once or twice daily. Promotes skin firmness, elasticity, and healing of photo-damaged skin.

KPV Peptide – 200–500 mcg subcutaneously or topically daily. Anti-inflammatory peptide that helps calm irritated or inflamed skin such as with eczema, dermatitis, or rosacea.

CJC-1295 with DAC + Ipamorelin – CJC-1295 with DAC 2 mg weekly + Ipamorelin 300 mcg daily. Stimulates GH/IGF-1 production and promotes skin thickness, healing, and youthful glow.

GHK-Cu + BPC-157 Topical Stack – blend both into a transdermal cream. Synergistically improves wound healing, reduces hyperpigmentation, and supports skin barrier repair.

LL-37 – 100–200 mcg subcutaneously near the skin lesion or orally daily. Antimicrobial peptide that aids in healing infected or chronic skin wounds.

Thymalin – 10–20 mg intramuscularly daily for 5–10 days. Restores thymic and skin tissue balance and supports regeneration and youthful skin structure.

Follistatin 344 – 100–300 mcg intramuscularly weekly for short cycles. It may assist in follicle regeneration and is being explored for reversing hair miniaturization.

DSIP (Delta Sleep-Inducing Peptide) – 100–200 mcg subcutaneously before bed. Improves deep sleep and cellular recovery, which enhances overnight skin repair.

Humanin (HNG) – 1–10 mg subcutaneously 2–3x per week. Reduces oxidative damage to skin and hair follicle cells. Slows signs of aging and supports resilience.

Chapter 13: 600 Protocols

Growth Hormone Secretagogue Stacks

1. **CJC-1295 with DAC + Ipamorelin** – Long-acting GH stimulation for muscle growth, fat loss, and recovery.

2. **CJC-1295 (no DAC) + GHRP-2** – Short-acting GH pulse ideal for multiple daily doses to maximize GH secretion.

3. **CJC-1295 (no DAC) + GHRP-6** – Promotes GH release and appetite stimulation. It is useful in bulking phases.

4. **CJC-1295 (no DAC) + Ipamorelin** – Lean muscle and fat-burning stack with minimal prolactin or cortisol side effects.

5. **Sermorelin + Ipamorelin** – Popular anti-aging and fat-burning stack. Improves sleep and recovery.

6. **Mod GRF 1-29 + Ipamorelin** – Pulsatile GH release with minimal desensitization. It is used for fat loss and lean mass gain.

7. **Mod GRF 1-29 + GHRP-2** – Ideal for body re-composition. Improves metabolic rate and sleep quality.

8. **Mod GRF 1-29 + GHRP-6** – Enhances appetite and GH output. It is used in recovery or muscle gain phases.

9. Tesamorelin + Ipamorelin – Visceral fat reduction and metabolic improvement, especially in older adults.

10. MK-677 (Ibutamoren) + CJC-1295 with DAC – Oral GH secretagogue with peptide support for enhanced body composition.

11. MK-677 + Ipamorelin – Synergistic boost in GH and IGF-1 for muscle hypertrophy and recovery.

12. MK-677 + Mod GRF 1-29 – Long- and short-acting stack for continuous GH elevation and pulsatile release.

13. MK-677 + GHRP-6 – Ideal for mass gaining with appetite support and GH optimization.

14. MK-677 + GHRP-2 – Boosts GH and supports fat loss with better appetite control than GHRP-6.

15. MK-677 + Tesamorelin – Enhances metabolic health, especially visceral fat reduction.

16. GHRP-2 + GHRH (CJC or GRF) – Classic GH pulse stack. Supports lean mass and skin health.

17. GHRP-6 + GHRH – Builds mass, boosts appetite, and supports joint recovery.

18. Ipamorelin + GHRH – Clean GH stack for fat loss and deep sleep support.

19. Tesamorelin + CJC-1295 – Advanced stack for abdominal fat loss and anti-aging.

20. GHRP-6 + GHRP-2 – Synergistic dual-ghrelin mimetic pulse. Promotes appetite and muscle repair.

21. GHRP-6 + Hexarelin – High GH output stack for size and recovery.

22. Ipamorelin + Hexarelin – Balances strong GH release with minimal prolactin spikes.

23. Ipamorelin + MK-677 – Long- and short-acting stack for 24-hour GH support.

24. MK-677 + GHRP-2 – Lean bulk protocol with improved sleep and recovery.

25. Hexarelin + CJC-1295 (no DAC) – Strong anabolic GH surge with potent pituitary stimulation.

26. MK-677 + GH Frag 176-191 – Boosts both GH and fat-burning effects synergistically.

27. Sermorelin + GH Frag 176-191 – Anti-aging and targeted fat-loss blend.

28. Ipamorelin + GH Frag 176-191 – Muscle preservation and localized fat loss.

29. Tesamorelin + GH Frag 176-191 – Abdominal fat reduction and improved insulin sensitivity.

30. CJC-1295 with DAC + GH Frag 176-191 – Long-term GH elevation and lipolysis for cutting.

31. CJC-1295 (no DAC) + MK-677 – Pulsatile GH with steady oral support for body re-composition.

32. Ipamorelin + AOD-9604 – Combines GH stimulation with fat-burning peptide for weight loss.

33. MK-677 + AOD-9604 – Oral and injectable stack to enhance fat metabolism and appetite control.

34. GHRP-2 + AOD-9604 – Supports GH release and targeted fat reduction.

35. CJC-1295 with DAC + AOD-9604 – Sustained GH release with fat-burning synergy.

36. Tesamorelin + AOD-9604 – Optimizes body fat loss and insulin regulation.

37. Sermorelin + AOD-9604 – Anti-aging stack for improved body composition.

38. Ipamorelin + Epitalon – Supports GH and pineal longevity. It is great for sleep and recovery.

39. MK-677 + Epitalon – Long-term health span optimization with GH and telomerase activity.

40. CJC-1295 with DAC + Epitalon – Full-body rejuvenation with hormonal and circadian support.

41. Tesamorelin + BPC-157 – Metabolic fat reduction with gut and tissue healing synergy.

42. MK-677 + BPC-157 – Combines GH axis stimulation with recovery and joint repair.

43. CJC-1295 + TB-500 – Enhances muscle growth and tissue regeneration simultaneously.

44. GHRP-2 + TB-500 – GH pulse with regenerative effects. It is ideal for athletes.

45. Hexarelin + BPC-157 – Heavy-duty healing and mass-building post-injury.

46. Sermorelin + Melanotan II – Combines GH benefits with libido and skin tone support.

47. CJC-1295 + Oxytocin – Hormonal balance and improved emotional wellness alongside GH support.

48. MK-677 + GHK-Cu – Anti-aging, hair and skin repair, and muscle preservation.

49. CJC-1295 + IGF-1 LR3 – GH-IGF-1 axis optimization for maximum muscle growth and recovery.

50. Ipamorelin + IGF-1 LR3 – Sustained GH release with direct IGF-1 effects for hypertrophy and fat metabolism.

Healing & Tissue Repair Combinations

1. **BPC-157 + TB-500** – Synergistic healing for muscles, tendons, ligaments, and joints.

2. **BPC-157 + GHK-Cu** – Accelerates skin regeneration and soft tissue healing.

3. **TB-500 + Thymosin Alpha-1** – Enhances immune-mediated tissue recovery and reduces systemic inflammation.

4. **BPC-157 + IGF-1 LR3** – Promotes muscle regeneration post-injury with anti-inflammatory support.

5. **BPC-157 + CJC-1295 + Ipamorelin** – Supports tissue repair through GH axis stimulation and localized healing.

6. **TB-500 + CJC-1295 with DAC + Ipamorelin** – Enhances muscle recovery, repair speed, and overall anabolism.

7. **BPC-157 + AOD-9604** – Supports tendon and joint healing. Reduces inflammation in fat pads or cartilage.

8. **TB-500 + GHK-Cu** – Enhances wound healing and angiogenesis in skin and connective tissue.

9. **BPC-157 + DSIP** – Accelerates healing by supporting restorative sleep and gut-brain repair axis.

10. BPC-157 + Epitalon – Anti-inflammatory and regenerative combination for long-term healing and tissue aging reversal.

11. BPC-157 + MOTS-c – Enhances mitochondrial-driven repair and cellular resilience in damaged tissues.

12. BPC-157 + LL-37 – Combats infection in chronic wounds and promotes tissue healing.

13. GHK-Cu + IGF-1 LR3 – Promotes soft tissue growth, skin repair, and collagen synthesis.

14. TB-500 + IGF-1 LR3 – Advanced stack for muscle regeneration and post-surgery or trauma recovery.

15. BPC-157 + KPV Peptide – Reduces inflammation and promotes healing in the gut, joints, and skin.

16. BPC-157 + Thymalin – Immune-regulated healing for autoimmune-related tissue damage.

17. TB-500 + BPC-157 + IGF-1 LR3 – Comprehensive healing protocol for severe injury or post-operative recovery.

18. BPC-157 + GHRP-2 + Mod GRF 1-29 – Enhances local repair and systemic GH-driven recovery.

19. TB-500 + GHRP-6 + CJC-1295 (no DAC) – Promotes appetite, GH release, and injury repair.

20. BPC-157 + NAD+ (IV or oral precursors) – Supports cellular energy needed for tissue repair and resilience.

21. TB-500 + Humanin – Mitochondrial protection during soft tissue regeneration and stress recovery.

22. GHK-Cu + BPC-157 + Epitalon – Advanced skin and tissue rejuvenation protocol with anti-aging synergy.

23. BPC-157 + Thymosin Beta-4 + KPV – Repairs epithelial damage, joint pain, and autoimmune-inflammation linked damage.

24. BPC-157 + Follistatin 344 – Enhances muscular regeneration and controls fibrosis.

25. TB-500 + Follistatin 344 – Promotes soft tissue recovery and muscle mass after immobilization or injury.

26. BPC-157 + Oxytocin (Peptide) – Speeds healing of soft tissues and supports pain relief through mood modulation.

27. TB-500 + Cerebrolysin – Aids neural and muscular regeneration post neurological trauma.

28. BPC-157 + Semax – Supports neurovascular repair and healing from brain or nerve injuries.

29. BPC-157 + MOTS-c + GHK-Cu – Skin, tendon, and joint repair stack with mitochondrial support.

30. BPC-157 + IGF-1 DES – Targets muscle healing and growth at injury sites.

31. BPC-157 + DSIP + TB-500 – Supports deep healing during restorative sleep for chronic injuries.

32. GHK-Cu + LL-37 – Ideal for wound care, tissue infections, and skin remodeling.

33. TB-500 + NAD+ + Humanin – Combines cellular repair and systemic anti-aging in post-trauma recovery.

34. BPC-157 + GHRH + GHRP Combination – Boosts GH axis and accelerates tendon and ligament recovery.

35. TB-500 + Epitalon + IGF-1 LR3 – Deep regenerative effects at cellular and tissue levels.

36. BPC-157 + SOD (Superoxide Dismutase Mimetics) – Reduces oxidative stress in joint and muscle healing.

37. GHK-Cu + CJC-1295 + Ipamorelin – Skin and collagen repair supported by GH elevation.

38. TB-500 + GHK-Cu + IGF-1 DES – Comprehensive skin, soft tissue, and muscle recovery.

39. BPC-157 + Semax + LL-37 – Nerve, gut, and soft tissue repair with antimicrobial benefits.

40. TB-500 + Mod GRF 1-29 + GHRP-6 – Enhances healing and GH release in trauma rehabilitation.

41. BPC-157 + Hyaluronic Acid Injections – Enhances joint repair and cartilage regeneration.

42. BPC-157 + AOD-9604 + TB-500 – Post-surgical recovery stack focused on mobility and healing.

43. BPC-157 + BDNF Mimetics – Supports neural repair and brain-body recovery after injury.

44. TB-500 + CJC-1295 + MK-677 – Maximizes muscle healing with long-acting GH release.

45. BPC-157 + Collagen Peptides (oral) – Supports structural regeneration of ligaments, tendons, and skin.

46. TB-500 + IGF-1 + MOTS-c – Combines GH/IGF repair with mitochondrial optimization for elite recovery.

47. BPC-157 + Rapamycin (low-dose) – Balances mTOR regulation with healing in age-related or chronic tissue damage.

48. BPC-157 + NR or NMN (NAD+ precursors) – Enhances recovery from chronic fatigue or connective tissue injury.

49. GHK-Cu + Thymalin + BPC-157 – Triple action skin and immune system healing combination.

50. TB-500 + GHK-Cu + DSIP – Repairs muscle and connective tissue during sleep cycles for optimal regeneration.

Nootropic & Cognitive Stacks

1. **Semax + Selank** – Enhances memory, focus, and reduces anxiety. Is great for cognitive enhancement under stress.

2. **Semax + Noopept** – Supports BDNF, neuroplasticity, and working memory for high cognitive demand tasks.

3. **Selank + Oxytocin** – Improves mood, sociability, and emotional processing in high-stress environments.

4. **Dihexa + Semax** – Strong neurogenic stack for long-term memory and synaptogenesis.

5. **Dihexa + Selank** – Supports neural repair and anxiety reduction. It is useful in trauma or cognitive burnout.

6. **Cerebrolysin + Semax** – Neurorestorative stack for memory loss, post-TBI, or age-related decline.

7. **Semax + DSIP** – Improves cognitive performance by combining daytime alertness with deeper sleep.

8. **Selank + DSIP** – Addresses anxiety-induced cognitive dysfunction and poor sleep recovery.

9. P21 + Dihexa – Advanced neuro-regenerative combination aimed at reversing memory impairment and neurodegeneration.

10. Cerebrolysin + P21 – Synergistic brain repair stack for neurotrauma and age-related cognitive issues.

11. MOTS-c + Semax – Mitochondrial energy and brain performance combination that is ideal for mental fatigue.

12. Humanin + Dihexa – Enhances cellular protection and neuroplasticity under oxidative stress.

13. Epitalon + Semax – Sleep and circadian support that improves long-term memory retention.

14. Semax + IGF-1 LR3 – Supports memory, nerve repair, and cognition in high-performance settings.

15. Selank + IGF-1 LR3 – Enhances learning and neural resilience, especially post-exam fatigue.

16. CJC-1295 + Ipamorelin + Semax – Combines GH support with BDNF activation for cognitive longevity.

17. Semax + L-Theanine – Smooths focus and reduces overstimulation. Ideal for high-anxiety performance.

18. Selank + Ashwagandha – Calms the nervous system and enhances cognitive control under chronic stress.

19. Dihexa + MOTS-c – Mitochondrial and synaptic repair combination to reverse cognitive fatigue.

20. Cerebrolysin + Epitalon – Brain anti-aging and circadian optimization for long-term cognitive health.

21. BDNF Mimetics + Dihexa – Promotes neuroplasticity and mental clarity for learning-intensive tasks.

22. GHK-Cu + Semax – Skin-brain anti-aging combination with neurotrophic and antioxidant effects.

23. P21 + Epitalon – Telomerase activation with brain regeneration. It is useful in neurodegenerative prevention.

24. Selank + Oxiracetam (oral) – Improves information processing speed, memory retention, and calmness.

25. Dihexa + Alpha-GPC – Boosts acetylcholine levels and neuron growth for sharp mental acuity.

26. MOTS-c + NAD+ Precursors (NR/NMN) – Supports brain energy, learning, and memory recall.

27. Cerebrolysin + NAD+ – Mitochondrial neurorepair stack for age-related cognitive decline.

28. Selank + Phenylpiracetam (oral) – Anxiety control with enhanced physical and mental performance.

29. Semax + N-Acetyl Selank – Improves focus, reduces fatigue, and enhances stress response.

30. Selank + PRL-8-53 (oral) – Short-term memory enhancement with reduced test anxiety.

31. Cerebrolysin + Dihexa + Semax – Full-spectrum neuroplasticity and brain repair protocol.

32. Semax + Lion's Mane Peptide – Supports BDNF and nerve growth factor synergistically.

33. Humanin + Epitalon + Selank – Cognitive longevity combination with mood and mitochondrial support.

34. DSIP + P21 – Deep sleep and regeneration stack to reverse cognitive overload.

35. GHK-Cu + Epitalon – Cellular repair with pineal gland support for neuroendocrine health.

36. Cerebrolysin + IGF-1 LR3 – Brain and nervous system recovery post-injury or concussion.

37. MOTS-c + BPC-157 – Gut-brain axis optimization for brain fog and systemic inflammation.

38. Dihexa + Fisetin (oral) – Synaptic regeneration with senolytic support to protect aging neurons.

39. Semax + Modafinil (oral) – Boosts alertness, cognition, and reduces fatigue in high-demand tasks.

40. Selank + CBD (oral/topical) – Anxiety, neuroinflammation, and cognition-support combination.

41. P21 + IGF-1 DES – Sharp synaptic regeneration in memory-focused protocols.

42. DSIP + Humanin – Improves sleep-based cognitive recovery and mitochondrial neuroprotection.

43. NAD+ + Dihexa + Semax – Ultimate mitochondrial and cognitive recovery stack.

44. Cerebrolysin + GHK-Cu – Anti-aging and neurotrophic peptide stack for cognitive enhancement.

45. Semax + Noopept + Alpha-GPC – High-performance memory and verbal fluency enhancer.

46. Lion's Mane Peptide + P21 – Combines NGF and neuro-regeneration for long-term cognitive benefit.

47. CJC-1295 + Epitalon + Semax – GH, pineal, and brain repair for aging-related brain decline.

48. Selank + Theobromine (oral) – Improves cerebral blood flow, mood, and alertness.

49. MOTS-c + DSIP + Semax – Mito-sleep-cognitive synergy for full brain performance recovery.

50. Humanin + P21 + NAD+ – Cognitive anti-aging stack to protect neurons and improve memory span.

Anti-Aging Synergy Stacks

1. **Epitalon + Thymalin** – Promotes immune rejuvenation and telomere restoration for lifespan extension.

2. **Epitalon + Pinealon** – Enhances circadian rhythm and cognitive longevity through pineal and brain peptides.

3. **CJC-1295 with DAC + Ipamorelin** – Sustains GH/IGF-1 for improved body composition, skin elasticity, and recovery.

4. **GHK-Cu + Epitalon** – Combines cellular rejuvenation with DNA repair and anti-wrinkle effects.

5. **Thymalin + GHK-Cu** – Stimulates collagen synthesis and thymic restoration for immune and skin health.

6. **Epitalon + MOTS-c** – Telomere repair plus mitochondrial enhancement for longevity support.

7. **MOTS-c + Humanin** – Mitochondrial synergy for stress resistance, metabolic support, and aging reversal.

8. **Epitalon + DSIP** – Enhances deep sleep, melatonin regulation, and nighttime cellular repair.

9. **GHK-Cu + Thymosin Beta-4 (TB-500)** – Full-body regenerative combination that targets tissue repair and skin quality.

10. Thymosin Alpha-1 + Epitalon – Immune resilience and anti-inflammatory peptide longevity stack.

11. CJC-1295 (no DAC) + GHRP-2 – Pulsatile GH release for anti-aging and metabolic balance.

12. CJC-1295 + IGF-1 LR3 – Improves lean body mass, skin firmness, and cognitive clarity.

13. MK-677 + Epitalon – GH secretagogue with circadian peptide for youthful hormone levels and sleep.

14. GHK-Cu + BPC-157 – Repairs connective tissues, skin, and gut lining for systemic anti-aging.

15. MOTS-c + NAD+ Precursors (NMN/NR) – Enhances mitochondrial and DNA repair for cellular longevity.

16. BPC-157 + KPV Peptide – Reduces chronic inflammation and promotes repair in joints and tissues.

17. Epitalon + IGF-1 LR3 – Supports skin, muscle, and hormone rejuvenation.

18. DSIP + GHRP-6 – Deep sleep and GH release synergy for nighttime recovery.

19. Semax + Epitalon – Enhances cognition, sleep, and pineal function to reduce cognitive aging.

20. Humanin + GHK-Cu – Repairs oxidative damage in the brain and skin to improve resilience and appearance.

21. NAD+ (IV or oral) + Epitalon – Telomere and mitochondrial combination for maximum anti-aging effect.

22. Thymalin + DSIP – Combines immune and endocrine support with enhanced deep restorative sleep.

23. CJC-1295 + TB-500 + Epitalon – GH support, tissue repair, and pineal rejuvenation in one stack.

24. GHK-Cu + IGF-1 LR3 – Boosts collagen, skin healing, and muscle regeneration.

25. MOTS-c + GHRH (CJC-1295) + BPC-157 – Mitochondrial health, GH balance, and gut-body healing.

26. Epitalon + LL-37 – Anti-aging immune balance and skin and wound antimicrobial protection.

27. GHK-Cu + MOTS-c – Skin, hair, and energy-boosting peptide combination.

28. BPC-157 + Epitalon + Thymalin – Supports anti-aging through tissue, immune, and endocrine harmony.

29. MK-677 + DSIP – Combines oral GH support with deep sleep optimization.

30. TB-500 + Epitalon + MOTS-c – Tissue regeneration, anti-inflammatory, and mitochondrial stack.

31. IGF-1 LR3 + Humanin – Enhances regeneration with neuroprotection and metabolic balance.

32. Semax + NAD+ Precursors – Improves brain energy and plasticity with anti-aging support.

33. CJC-1295 with DAC + AOD-9604 – GH modulation with fat metabolism improvement in aging adults.

34. Thymalin + MOTS-c – Immune regeneration and mitochondrial support for healthy aging.

35. Epitalon + GHK-Cu + DSIP – Deep restoration of circadian, tissue, and skin function.

36. KPV Peptide + TB-500 – Anti-inflammatory and regenerative blend for autoimmune aging cases.

37. NAD+ + Humanin + MOTS-c – Mitochondrial longevity trinity for age-related energy decline.

38. GHK-Cu + Hyaluronic Acid (topical/IM) – Skin rejuvenation, moisture retention, and wrinkle reduction.

39. Epitalon + CJC-1295 + Ipamorelin – Youthful hormonal profile and pineal repair synergy.

40. Dihexa + Semax + Epitalon – Brain enhancement, plasticity, and circadian rhythm restoration.

41. BPC-157 + IGF-1 LR3 + NAD+ – Repair stack for high-performance aging and injury recovery.

42. GHK-Cu + BPC-157 + TB-500 – Joint and skin rejuvenation for physically active aging adults.

43. GHRH + GHRP-6 + Epitalon – GH, appetite, and pineal hormone synergy for anti-aging.

44. GHK-Cu + DSIP + Thymalin – Skin healing, sleep regulation, and immune resetting for longevity.

45. Semax + MOTS-c – Focus, energy, and resilience combination against cognitive and metabolic aging.

46. MK-677 + Epitalon + Thymalin – Oral GH boost with hormonal and immune rejuvenation.

47. CJC-1295 + BPC-157 + GHK-Cu – GH support and connective tissue rejuvenation in a holistic aging stack.

48. Thymosin Alpha-1 + KPV Peptide – Systemic immune modulation and anti-inflammatory synergy.

49. GHK-Cu + Collagen Peptides (oral) – Improves elasticity, joint health, and anti-wrinkle effects.

50. Epitalon + DSIP + MOTS-c – Core anti-aging sleep, mitochondrial, and pineal optimization trio.

Fat Loss & Metabolic Optimization

1. **AOD-9604 + CJC-1295 with DAC** – Enhances lipolysis and boosts GH levels for fat-burning and lean muscle retention.

2. **HGH Frag 176-191 + Ipamorelin** – Potent fat-burning combination with minimal GH-related side effects.

3. **Tesamorelin + AOD-9604** – Synergistic visceral fat reduction. It is particularly effective in abdominal obesity.

4. **CJC-1295 (no DAC) + GHRP-2 + AOD-9604** – Pulsatile GH release for fat loss with increased metabolism and reduced fat storage.

5. **MK-677 + AOD-9604** – Supports fat burning and improves recovery with oral convenience.

6. **Tesamorelin + GHRP-2** – GH axis optimization for fat loss and insulin sensitivity.

7. **HGH Frag 176-191 + AOD-9604** – Double-fragment stack for advanced adipose tissue targeting.

8. **MOTS-c + AOD-9604** – Mitochondrial metabolic support combined with fat-specific lipopeptide.

9. **CJC-1295 + Ipamorelin + AOD-9604** – Powerful metabolic-enhancing combination with synergistic fat-burning.

10. 5-Amino-1MQ + MOTS-c – NNMT and mitochondrial targeting for increased basal metabolic rate and fat oxidation.

11. 5-Amino-1MQ + Tesofensine – Boosts metabolism and suppresses appetite for rapid body fat reduction.

12. Tesofensine + AOD-9604 – Appetite suppression and direct lipolysis in a cutting phase protocol.

13. 5-Amino-1MQ + CJC-1295 + Ipamorelin – Advanced fat loss stack that targets both hormonal and metabolic levers.

14. MOTS-c + Humanin – Mitochondrial peptide synergy for metabolic health and weight control.

15. Semaglutide + AOD-9604 – Appetite control with direct fat loss activation.

16. Tesamorelin + MOTS-c – Visceral fat reduction with improved insulin signaling.

17. 5-Amino-1MQ + MK-677 – Muscle-preserving fat loss with metabolic acceleration.

18. Tesofensine + MOTS-c – Thermogenic combination with appetite suppression and enhanced energy utilization.

19. HGH Frag 176-191 + 5-Amino-1MQ – Lipolytic peptide stack with NNMT inhibition for stubborn fat.

20. CJC-1295 + GH Frag 176-191 + MOTS-c – Hormonal and mitochondrial fat-burning triple stack.

21. GHRP-6 + Mod GRF 1-29 + AOD-9604 – Appetite regulation with GH-mediated lipolysis.

22. CJC-1295 (no DAC) + GH Frag 176-191 – Optimized fat loss without GH side effects.

23. MK-677 + GH Frag 176-191 – Oral GH secretagogue with localized fat loss synergy.

24. BPC-157 + AOD-9604 – Joint-gut repair with enhanced mobility and fat metabolism.

25. MOTS-c + NAD+ Precursors (NMN/NR) – Mitochondrial rejuvenation and improved fat oxidation.

26. Tesamorelin + NAD+ IV or oral – Enhanced mitochondrial metabolism and GH support.

27. CJC-1295 with DAC + Tesofensine – Long-acting GH stimulation with powerful appetite suppressant.

28. GH Frag 176-191 + KPV Peptide – Reduces inflammation-driven fat accumulation and metabolic dysfunction.

29. AOD-9604 + KPV Peptide – Combines fat loss and anti-inflammatory activity in obese or metabolic syndrome patients.

30. 5-Amino-1MQ + NAD+ – Cellular energy enhancement and metabolism boost for resistant fat loss.

31. MOTS-c + Epitalon – Circadian-metabolic fat loss enhancer with anti-aging synergy.

32. Semaglutide + MOTS-c – GLP-1 and mitochondrial synergy for enhanced glucose and fat metabolism.

33. Tesofensine + GHRP-2 – Appetite control and GH release to preserve lean mass during fat loss.

34. Tesamorelin + 5-Amino-1MQ – Visceral fat reduction with enhanced mitochondrial lipid oxidation.

35. Tesamorelin + CJC-1295 – Double GHRH stack for aggressive GH secretion and abdominal fat targeting.

36. MOTS-c + CJC-1295 + Ipamorelin – Full-spectrum GH and mitochondrial synergy for fat loss and endurance.

37. GH Frag 176-191 + Semaglutide – Lipolysis and appetite regulation with minimal muscle loss.

38. Tesamorelin + Epitalon – Improves GH output and regulates circadian metabolic balance.

39. MK-677 + Semaglutide – Muscle-sparing GH boost with GLP-1 fat loss and appetite control.

40. GHRP-2 + GH Frag 176-191 + Tesamorelin – Multi-angled GH-based fat loss protocol.

41. GH Frag 176-191 + Humanin – Mitochondrial protection and fat loss during calorie deficits.

42. KPV Peptide + MOTS-c – Anti-inflammatory metabolic enhancer for insulin resistance and belly fat.

43. Tesofensine + MK-677 – Fat loss and muscle support with stimulant-free energy increase.

44. GHK-Cu + AOD-9604 – Skin rejuvenation with fat reduction and healing in cosmetic fat loss protocols.

45. TB-500 + AOD-9604 – Recovery and mobility support in fat-loss focused athletes.

46. CJC-1295 + AOD-9604 + Semaglutide – Full-spectrum metabolic control with hormonal and satiety modulation.

47. BPC-157 + MOTS-c – Gut-brain axis healing with mitochondrial fat metabolism support.

48. Epitalon + AOD-9604 – Fat metabolism support through circadian and pineal rejuvenation.

49. Tesofensine + Humanin – Appetite suppression plus mitochondrial stress protection.

50. Semaglutide + 5-Amino-1MQ – One of the most aggressive metabolic stacks for rapid, medically monitored weight loss.

Libido, Performance, & Sexual Health

1. PT-141 (Bremelanotide) + Oxytocin – Boosts libido and emotional bonding. Enhances arousal and orgasm response in both sexes.

2. Melanotan II (low dose) + PT-141 – Synergistic effect on sexual arousal, spontaneous erections, and increased desire.

3. Kisspeptin-10 + Gonadorelin – Enhances natural testosterone and LH production for improved libido and fertility.

4. CJC-1295 with DAC + Ipamorelin + PT-141 – Combines GH support with increased libido and erectile function.

5. PT-141 + DSIP – Enhances arousal and improves sleep quality and hormonal recovery.

6. Melanotan II + Oxytocin – Enhances emotional intimacy and sexual drive, with added tanning effects.

7. PT-141 + GHK-Cu – Improves sexual responsiveness and vascularity with skin and hair health support.

8. Oxytocin + GHRP-2 – Boosts mood and testosterone through the GH axis. Supports libido under stress.

9. BPC-157 + PT-141 – Aids erectile tissue healing post-injury and enhances sexual performance.

10. IGF-1 LR3 + PT-141 – Enhances tissue regeneration, stamina, and arousal response.

11. MK-677 + Oxytocin – Increases growth hormone and emotional bonding. Improves libido and sleep.

12. Humanin + PT-141 – Combats fatigue and mitochondrial dysfunction which impact sexual performance.

13. Tesamorelin + PT-141 – Fat loss and libido enhancement. It is ideal for overweight individuals with low libido.

14. 5-Amino-1MQ + PT-141 – Improves metabolism and energy for better sexual endurance and fat loss.

15. Semax + PT-141 – Enhances mental clarity, mood, and sexual desire in high-stress individuals.

16. BPC-157 + TB-500 + PT-141 – Improves vascular and soft tissue health. It is great for erectile recovery protocols.

17. CJC-1295 + Oxytocin + PT-141 – Enhances hormone balance, intimacy, and full sexual function.

18. MOTS-c + PT-141 – Improves endurance and metabolic health for high-functioning sexual energy.

19. PT-141 + NAD+ (IV or oral) – Supports mitochondrial libido and stamina in aging individuals.

20. Follistatin 344 + PT-141 – Myostatin inhibition for lean mass and libido synergy.

21. Epitalon + Oxytocin – Supports mood, sleep, and libido with anti-aging endocrine support.

22. GHK-Cu + Oxytocin – Enhances bonding, sexual wellness, and skin and hair health.

23. PT-141 + Semaglutide – Addresses libido in individuals undergoing GLP-1-based weight loss.

24. Thymalin + Oxytocin – Restores endocrine health, sexual motivation, and emotional balance.

25. Dihexa + PT-141 – Enhances arousal and neural connections associated with intimacy and desire.

26. MK-677 + PT-141 – Increases GH and libido, and promotes lean muscle and endurance.

27. GHRP-6 + PT-141 – Appetite and libido stimulation for bulking or low-libido states.

28. TB-500 + Oxytocin – Combines healing and emotional support for intimacy restoration post-injury or trauma.

29. Kisspeptin-10 + PT-141 – Boosts natural testosterone and sexual arousal.

30. DSIP + Oxytocin – Sleep and intimacy enhancer. It is useful in stress-induced sexual dysfunction.

31. Melanotan II + Humanin – Enhances arousal and reduces fatigue in older adults.

32. GHK-Cu + BPC-157 + PT-141 – Erectile tissue regeneration and libido boost post-surgery or damage.

33. Tesofensine + PT-141 – Weight loss and arousal enhancer in obese or metabolically suppressed individuals.

34. IGF-1 DES + PT-141 – Promotes localized tissue growth and recovery in the genital region.

35. Semax + Oxytocin – Combines mental clarity, emotional bonding, and sex drive enhancement.

36. MOTS-c + NAD+ + PT-141 – Cellular energy and libido booster stack for age-related decline.

37. CJC-1295 with DAC + PT-141 + Oxytocin – Hormonal balance, sexual vigor, and intimacy protocol.

38. 5-Amino-1MQ + Oxytocin – Mood and metabolism support for low-libido caused by depression or fatigue.

39. GHRP-2 + Oxytocin + Semax – Multifactorial approach to enhance libido, testosterone, and mental engagement.

40. Epitalon + PT-141 – Anti-aging and libido rejuvenation stack. It is ideal for perimenopause or andropause.

41. LL-37 + BPC-157 + PT-141 – Supports urogenital healing and combats low libido linked to chronic infections.

42. GHK-Cu + CJC-1295 + PT-141 – Skin and hair regeneration with sexual performance boost.

43. DSIP + PT-141 + Thymalin – Sleep, hormone regulation, and libido stack for older individuals.

44. MK-677 + Oxytocin + BPC-157 – Long-term healing and intimacy enhancement combination.

45. PT-141 + Lion's Mane Peptide (experimental) – Enhances arousal and sensory processing for sexual connection.

46. Kisspeptin + CJC-1295 + PT-141 – Triple-hormone enhancer for performance, libido, and fertility.

47. Tesamorelin + Oxytocin + BPC-157 – Metabolic, emotional, and physical intimacy support.

48. GHRP-2 + Epitalon + PT-141 – GH secretion, pineal rejuvenation, and sexual motivation.

49. 5-Amino-1MQ + GHRP-6 + PT-141 – Energy, appetite, and libido restoration in metabolic burnout.

50. Semax + DSIP + PT-141 – Combines daytime mental clarity, deep sleep, and peak arousal.

Immune & Autoimmune Regulation Stacks

1. Thymosin Alpha-1 + Thymalin – Enhances T-cell function and restores immune system balance in autoimmune and chronic infections.

2. BPC-157 + KPV Peptide – Reduces gut and systemic inflammation. It is ideal for IBD, leaky gut, and autoimmune flare prevention.

3. Thymosin Alpha-1 + LL-37 – Immune activation and antimicrobial defense for chronic viral or bacterial infections.

4. KPV + TB-500 – Anti-inflammatory and tissue repair combination for autoimmunity with joint-muscle damage.

5. BPC-157 + TB-500 – Combines gut healing with systemic soft tissue repair. It is useful in autoimmune musculoskeletal disorders.

6. GHK-Cu + Thymalin – Restores immune homeostasis and tissue repair in age-related immune decline.

7. Epitalon + Thymalin – Immune-pineal axis reset for autoimmune disease and immune rejuvenation.

8. Thymosin Alpha-1 + DSIP – Enhances immune recovery and sleep-dependent cytokine balance.

9. LL-37 + BPC-157 – Mucosal barrier healing with antimicrobial activity in chronic infection-related autoimmunity.

10. KPV + Epitalon – Reduces inflammation and supports immune regulation through circadian balance.

11. MOTS-c + Thymosin Alpha-1 – Improves mitochondrial-driven immune resilience in chronic fatigue syndromes.

12. NAD+ + Thymalin – Supports immune cell energy metabolism in immune-compromised individuals.

13. Selank + Thymosin Alpha-1 – Reduces neuroinflammation and immune dysregulation triggered by stress.

14. GHK-Cu + KPV – Skin and mucosal immune support for eczema, psoriasis, or dermatitis-related autoimmunity.

15. Thymalin + BPC-157 – Autoimmune balancing with epithelial repair for gut and skin conditions.

16. Humanin + KPV Peptide – Mitochondrial peptide that helps reduce oxidative immune damage in autoimmunity.

17. Epitalon + Thymosin Alpha-1 – Telomerase and immune restoration stack for chronic inflammatory diseases.

18. TB-500 + LL-37 – Repairs tissue and modulates infection-related inflammation.

19. Thymalin + MOTS-c – Boosts immune tolerance and reduces auto-reactivity through mitochondrial-immune axis.

20. BPC-157 + Semax – Gut-brain-immune axis support for post-viral fatigue and stress-related immune imbalance.

21. KPV Peptide + Selank – CNS-immune calming protocol for anxiety-triggered autoimmune flares.

22. Thymosin Alpha-1 + BPC-157 + KPV – Triple-action immune, epithelial, and anti-inflammatory regulation.

23. DSIP + Thymalin – Enhances sleep and thymic output for autoimmunity driven by poor regeneration.

24. LL-37 + Epitalon – Combats immune senescence and chronic infection-triggered autoimmunity.

25. Thymalin + GHK-Cu + NAD+ – Aging immune restoration with mitochondrial energy and skin-mucosal support.

26. KPV + MOTS-c – Lowers inflammation and improves insulin sensitivity in metabolic-autoimmune overlap.

27. BPC-157 + IGF-1 LR3 – Tissue recovery and inflammation modulation for autoimmune myopathy or fibromyalgia.

28. Thymosin Alpha-1 + CJC-1295 – Enhances immunity and GH-induced cellular repair in long COVID or chronic infection.

29. Epitalon + DSIP + Thymalin – Complete circadian-immune reset for autoimmune disease progression control.

30. LL-37 + GHK-Cu – Antimicrobial peptide with copper peptide to support skin and respiratory immunity.

31. KPV Peptide + GHRP-2 – Reduces inflammation and modulates the GH-immune axis. It is useful in autoimmunity with catabolism.

32. BPC-157 + KPV + IGF-1 LR3 – Gut-skin-muscle repair combination for autoimmune syndromes with tissue breakdown.

33. Selank + BPC-157 – Gut-brain immune harmonization for neuroinflammatory and gut-autoimmune overlap such as in MS or IBS.

34. Humanin + Epitalon – Mitochondrial and pineal peptide pair for aging immune dysfunction and oxidative stress.

35. Thymosin Beta-4 + KPV – Repair of connective tissue and modulation of inflammatory pathways in autoimmunity.

36. NAD+ + MOTS-c + Thymalin – Energizes immune cell function and reduces chronic immune activation.

37. GHK-Cu + LL-37 + BPC-157 – Wound and immune barrier repair, especially for skin-dominant autoimmune conditions.

38. TB-500 + KPV + Humanin – Combines tissue regeneration, inflammation reduction, and cellular protection.

39. BPC-157 + CJC-1295 + Thymalin – GH, gut repair, and thymic renewal stack for autoimmune recovery.

40. Thymosin Alpha-1 + IGF-1 LR3 – Immune modulation with anabolic support for autoimmune muscle loss.

41. KPV + GHK-Cu + DSIP – Anti-inflammatory and skin-brain axis restoration with sleep regulation.

42. Semax + Thymalin – Brain-immune support for post-viral syndromes and neuro-autoimmune disorders.

43. TB-500 + MOTS-c + NAD+ – Regenerative and metabolic support for immune-mediated degenerative diseases.

44. LL-37 + Thymosin Alpha-1 + Epitalon – Viral defense and immune aging control for frequent infections.

45. KPV Peptide + NAD+ Precursors (NR/NMN) – Cellular inflammation reduction and energy restoration in immune burnout.

46. BPC-157 + KPV + DSIP – Gut-immune-sleep optimization for flares triggered by circadian disruption.

47. Thymalin + Humanin – Mitochondrial and thymic repair for aging-related autoimmunity.

48. LL-37 + TB-500 + MOTS-c – Combats infection-driven inflammation in autoimmune disease recovery.

49. GHK-Cu + Epitalon + Thymosin Alpha-1 – Reverses immune aging and supports cellular balance.

50. Selank + Thymalin + BPC-157 – Neurological, immune, and gastrointestinal regulation for stress-induced immune imbalance.

Gut & GI Healing Stacks

1. **BPC-157 + KPV Peptide** – Potent anti-inflammatory and mucosal healing combination for leaky gut and IBD.

2. **BPC-157 + TB-500** – Supports epithelial regeneration and connective tissue healing in chronic gut injury.

3. **BPC-157 + GHK-Cu** – Enhances gut lining repair and collagen regeneration in ulcerative or inflamed GI tracts.

4. **BPC-157 + LL-37** – Combines barrier healing with antimicrobial defense in SIBO and chronic GI infections.

5. **KPV Peptide + LL-37** – Immune and antimicrobial modulation for colitis, SIBO, and gut dysbiosis.

6. **BPC-157 + Epitalon** – Restores circadian rhythm and intestinal regeneration in gut-brain axis disorders.

7. **BPC-157 + DSIP** – Supports GI recovery through enhanced deep sleep and anti-stress pathways.

8. **KPV Peptide + DSIP** – Calms inflammation and improves gut motility through stress-hormone regulation.

9. BPC-157 + NAD+ Precursors (NR/NMN) – Enhances cellular repair and energy metabolism in inflamed gut tissue.

10. TB-500 + BPC-157 + KPV – Triple-action gut regeneration and inflammation control for severe IBD cases.

11. LL-37 + BPC-157 + TB-500 – Advanced antimicrobial and epithelial support for long-standing gut infection or ulceration.

12. Thymosin Alpha-1 + BPC-157 – Immune tolerance and gut lining support in autoimmunity-linked GI disorders.

13. Thymalin + BPC-157 – Endocrine-immune support for gut repair in stress-induced gut permeability.

14. MOTS-c + BPC-157 – Mitochondrial resilience and mucosal repair. It is great for fatigue and GI inflammation.

15. KPV + GHK-Cu – Anti-inflammatory and regenerative combination for epithelial barrier integrity.

16. BPC-157 + GHRP-2 – Enhances GI healing through gut-specific growth hormone release.

17. Epitalon + KPV Peptide – Circadian and anti-inflammatory synergy for gut lining and microbiome balance.

18. LL-37 + KPV Peptide + NAD+ – Antimicrobial, inflammation-reducing, and cellular repair for GI dysbiosis and leaky gut.

19. TB-500 + KPV Peptide – Tissue and epithelial healing for post-surgical gut repair or long-term inflammation.

20. BPC-157 + Humanin – Protects the gut from oxidative stress and supports mitochondrial integrity.

21. DSIP + BPC-157 + NAD+ – Deep healing during sleep with energy metabolism for long-term gut damage repair.

22. GHK-Cu + LL-37 – Promotes antimicrobial defense and mucosal rejuvenation for GERD and colitis.

23. Thymalin + KPV Peptide – Immune tolerance and anti-inflammatory combination for autoimmunity-related gut symptoms.

24. BPC-157 + IGF-1 LR3 – Epithelial regeneration and anabolic repair for bowel wall recovery.

25. KPV Peptide + Oxytocin – Gut-brain calming combination to support vagal tone and GI motility.

26. MOTS-c + KPV Peptide – Enhances insulin sensitivity and gut inflammation modulation in metabolic-gut syndrome.

27. BPC-157 + TB-500 + Epitalon – Total-body regenerative gut repair for inflammatory and aging-related GI decline.

28. LL-37 + NAD+ – Antimicrobial mucosal defense with cellular energy support for gut tissue healing.

29. Semax + BPC-157 – Supports gut-brain axis, especially in gut-induced brain fog or mood dysfunction.

30. KPV Peptide + DSIP + Thymalin – Deep healing protocol for sleep-driven immune-gut regeneration.

31. BPC-157 + Collagen Peptides (oral) – Supports collagen matrix and epithelial lining in gut wall restoration.

32. GHK-Cu + BPC-157 + DSIP – Skin-gut barrier recovery and sleep-enhanced GI repair.

33. TB-500 + GHK-Cu + BPC-157 – Epithelial and connective tissue healing for severe colitis or gastritis.

34. BPC-157 + Probiotic Therapy – Synergistic approach to microbiome and gut lining regeneration.

35. LL-37 + Humanin + KPV – Combats infection and oxidative stress and restores epithelial immunity.

36. BPC-157 + KPV + Semaglutide (low dose) – Aids weight loss and gut health in metabolic-gut inflammation.

37. NAD+ + BPC-157 + Epitalon – Mitochondrial and circadian repair for gut wall dysfunction.

38. Thymosin Alpha-1 + GHK-Cu – Immune modulation and repair in food sensitivity and chronic GI inflammation.

39. BPC-157 + TB-500 + IGF-1 LR3 – Accelerated recovery for intestinal surgery or Crohn's flare repair.

40. KPV Peptide + Alpha-Lipoic Acid (oral) – Antioxidant-enhanced mucosal recovery and inflammation control.

41. MOTS-c + BPC-157 + LL-37 – Mitochondrial and microbial repair combination for post-antibiotic gut syndrome.

42. DSIP + LL-37 + Thymalin – Sleep-driven mucosal repair and immune tolerance stack.

43. BPC-157 + Thymalin + GHK-Cu – Advanced mucosal, immune, and skin-gut axis healing.

44. Epitalon + NAD+ + BPC-157 – Anti-aging protocol for GI lining and digestive enzyme regulation.

45. KPV Peptide + NMN/NR (oral) – Mitochondrial inflammation control and gut-brain regulation.

46. BPC-157 + Oxytocin + KPV – Vagal tone, mucosal recovery, and GI inflammation reduction for IBS.

47. GHK-Cu + LL-37 + NAD+ – Cellular regeneration and antimicrobial repair in persistent gut dysbiosis.

48. BPC-157 + DSIP + MOTS-c – Nighttime gut healing with mitochondrial recovery for GI burnout.

49. Thymalin + LL-37 + KPV Peptide – Immune regulation and pathogen control in gut autoimmunity.

50. BPC-157 + CJC-1295 + KPV Peptide – GH support with gut lining and inflammation modulation for weight-loss or aging-related GI repair.

Sleep & Recovery Stacks

1. **DSIP + Epitalon** – Enhances deep sleep and circadian rhythm for full-body recovery.

2. **DSIP + BPC-157** – Promotes sleep quality and soft tissue regeneration during rest.

3. **DSIP + TB-500** – Sleep-enhanced muscle, tendon, and ligament repair.

4. **DSIP + IGF-1 LR3** – Improves deep recovery post-training by boosting anabolic signaling during sleep.

5. **DSIP + CJC-1295 with DAC + Ipamorelin** – Supports GH release during sleep for physical and cognitive recovery.

6. **DSIP + GHK-Cu** – Accelerates skin and soft tissue recovery and improves sleep quality.

7. **DSIP + KPV Peptide** – Reduces inflammation and improves healing in inflammatory sleep disorders.

8. **DSIP + NAD+ (IV or oral)** – Enhances mitochondrial sleep recovery and cellular energy replenishment.

9. **DSIP + MOTS-c** – Supports restorative mitochondrial repair during sleep in aging or high-stress individuals.

10. DSIP + Humanin – Protects neurons and organs from oxidative stress overnight.

11. DSIP + Thymalin – Deep immune and endocrine rejuvenation through enhanced sleep.

12. DSIP + Semax – Cognitive restoration and mental clarity enhancement after sleep.

13. DSIP + Oxytocin – Balances emotional processing and sleep quality in trauma recovery.

14. DSIP + Epitalon + NAD+ – Anti-aging and circadian stack for elite recovery and longevity.

15. DSIP + BPC-157 + TB-500 – Advanced recovery stack for musculoskeletal and gut healing during sleep.

16. DSIP + GHRP-2 + CJC-1295 (no DAC) – Pulsatile GH stimulation overnight for enhanced muscle and tissue repair.

17. Epitalon + BPC-157 – Circadian repair and gastrointestinal recovery synergy during nighttime cycles.

18. Epitalon + Semax – Pineal support and neuro-regeneration when asleep.

19. DSIP + GHK-Cu + NAD+ – Mitochondrial, anti-inflammatory, and tissue recovery optimization.

20. DSIP + IGF-1 DES – Localized tissue regeneration paired with deep systemic recovery.

21. DSIP + KPV + TB-500 – Inflammation resolution and joint-tendon healing with restful sleep.

22. DSIP + LL-37 – Sleep-enhanced immune response and microbial defense.

23. DSIP + Selank – Stress reduction and GABAergic sleep improvement in anxiety-related insomnia.

24. DSIP + GHRP-6 + Mod GRF 1-29 – Optimizes GH pulses and enhances recovery through deep sleep.

25. DSIP + MOTS-c + Humanin – Cellular energy and neuroimmune resilience during sleep.

26. DSIP + 5-Amino-1MQ – Metabolic recovery enhancement in sleep for athletes or weight loss.

27. DSIP + IGF-1 LR3 + Epitalon – Elite anti-aging recovery protocol combining GH, IGF, and pineal optimization.

28. DSIP + BPC-157 + NAD+ – Gut-brain repair and mitochondrial restoration overnight.

29. DSIP + TB-500 + CJC-1295 (no DAC) – Repair-focused recovery stack for muscle and joint healing.

30. DSIP + Humanin + Epitalon – Mitochondrial and endocrine harmony with deep sleep and aging support.

31. DSIP + Thymosin Alpha-1 – Immune tolerance, sleep regulation, and recovery from immune stress.

32. DSIP + IGF-1 LR3 + KPV Peptide – Combines inflammation control and anabolic recovery in sleep cycles.

33. DSIP + MOTS-c + NAD+ Precursors (NR/NMN) – Comprehensive mitochondrial and hormonal sleep repair.

34. DSIP + Follistatin 344 – Muscle regeneration and hormonal optimization during deep sleep.

35. DSIP + LL-37 + BPC-157 – Combines gut, immune, and soft tissue repair during sleep.

36. DSIP + Semax + GHK-Cu – Brain and skin recovery stack ideal for post-stress rejuvenation.

37. DSIP + Epitalon + Thymalin – Complete neuroendocrine anti-aging recovery protocol.

38. DSIP + TB-500 + IGF-1 LR3 – Powerful tissue repair for athletes or post-injury healing.

39. DSIP + CJC-1295 with DAC + NAD+ – Deep GH release with mitochondrial repair support.

40. DSIP + Selank + Epitalon – Enhances mood stability and pineal support with restful sleep.

41. DSIP + BPC-157 + LL-37 – GI and mucosal repair combined with immune recovery during sleep.

42. DSIP + GHK-Cu + TB-500 – Soft tissue healing with deep regenerative sleep benefit.

43. DSIP + CJC-1295 + IGF-1 LR3 – Full recovery stack for strength athletes during off-cycle.

44. DSIP + Oxytocin + Epitalon – Balances emotional and hormonal cycles during nighttime repair.

45. DSIP + Semax + KPV Peptide – Brain inflammation reduction and improved memory through restful sleep.

46. DSIP + NAD+ + MOTS-c – Metabolic night repair for long-term mitochondrial fatigue.

47. DSIP + MK-677 – Oral GH mimic combined with sleep-induced recovery for ease and convenience.

48. DSIP + GHRH + GHRP-2 – Balanced GH release and sleep synergy in aging adults.

49. DSIP + Humanin + GHK-Cu – Mitochondrial and skin repair overnight with neurological protection.

50. DSIP + Epitalon + Selank + NAD+ – Ultimate anti-aging and recovery protocol for elite performers.

Skin & Hair Rejuvenation Stacks

1. GHK-Cu + BPC-157 – Accelerates skin repair, reduces scarring, and improves elasticity and hydration.

2. GHK-Cu + TB-500 – Supports dermal tissue regeneration, especially in stretch marks or aged skin.

3. GHK-Cu + Epitalon – Combines anti-aging gene expression with collagen and skin rejuvenation.

4. GHK-Cu + IGF-1 LR3 – Promotes collagen synthesis and scalp circulation for skin firmness and hair follicle growth.

5. GHK-Cu + CJC-1295 with DAC + Ipamorelin – Improves skin tone and hair health through GH/IGF-1 stimulation.

6. GHK-Cu + MOTS-c – Enhances mitochondrial energy and antioxidant effects for youthful skin.

7. GHK-Cu + NAD+ (IV or topical precursor) – Repairs DNA damage, reduces fine lines, and improves skin cell turnover.

8. GHK-Cu + LL-37 – Promotes wound healing and antimicrobial skin protection in acne and damaged skin.

9. GHK-Cu + Hyaluronic Acid (topical) – Boosts moisture retention and skin plumpness in dry or aging skin.

10. GHK-Cu + Oxytocin (topical or subQ) – Enhances skin glow and texture through increased circulation and bonding.

11. BPC-157 + TB-500 – Deep tissue and dermal regeneration for chronic skin injuries and scars.

12. GHK-Cu + Copper Peptides (topical stack) – Combines systemic and local delivery to rebuild damaged or aged skin.

13. GHK-Cu + Follistatin 344 – Potential support for hair follicle enlargement and scalp restoration.

14. IGF-1 LR3 + GHK-Cu (scalp injections) – Promotes hair thickening and follicular repair in androgenic alopecia.

15. GHK-Cu + KPV Peptide – Reduces skin inflammation and stimulates collagen and regeneration.

16. BPC-157 + GHK-Cu + Epitalon – Comprehensive anti-aging skin protocol addressing DNA repair, elasticity, and tone.

17. GHK-Cu + TB-500 + LL-37 – Skin integrity and immunity boost for eczema, rosacea, or psoriasis.

18. GHK-Cu + BPC-157 + DSIP – Enhances nighttime skin healing and rejuvenation.

19. GHK-Cu + GHRP-6 + CJC-1295 (no DAC) – Boosts growth hormone for skin repair and smoothness.

20. GHK-Cu + AOD-9604 – Reduces localized fat deposits in the face and neck and enhances skin tone.

21. IGF-1 LR3 + DSIP – Combines tissue regeneration and deep sleep-driven recovery for skin cell turnover.

22. GHK-Cu + C60 (topical or oral antioxidant) – Reduces oxidative aging and supports DNA repair in skin cells.

23. GHK-Cu + Epitalon + MOTS-c – Anti-aging stack that supports mitochondrial and dermal rejuvenation.

24. GHK-Cu + Semax – Enhances skin-brain connection and antioxidant regeneration in neurogenic skin disorders.

25. GHK-Cu + LL-37 + Hyaluronic Acid – Moisture, antimicrobial, and healing stack for sensitive or damaged skin.

26. GHK-Cu + NMN (oral or topical) – Activates NAD+ pathways for cellular skin repair and wrinkle reduction.

27. GHK-Cu + BPC-157 + Semaglutide (low dose) – Aesthetic combination for weight loss with skin tightening support.

28. GHK-Cu + IGF-1 DES (topical/scalp) – Targeted support for hair follicle cycling and dermal regeneration.

29. GHK-Cu + Fisetin (oral senolytic) – Combats senescent skin cells to promote a youthful glow.

30. GHK-Cu + MOTS-c + NAD+ – Full mitochondrial and collagen repair stack for skin aging reversal.

31. GHK-Cu + Vitamin C Serum (topical) – Enhances collagen crosslinking and brightens complexion.

32. GHK-Cu + CJC-1295 + IGF-1 LR3 – GH axis and copper synergy to rejuvenate aging skin and scalp.

33. GHK-Cu + Retinoic Acid (topical) – Potentiates cell turnover and reduces pigmentation.

34. GHK-Cu + BPC-157 + LL-37 – Antimicrobial and skin-barrier repair protocol for acne-prone skin.

35. GHK-Cu + Rapamycin (topical microdose) – Combats skin senescence and aging through mTOR modulation.

36. GHK-Cu + TB-500 + Epitalon – Regenerates connective tissue and promotes youthful dermal structure.

37. GHK-Cu + Thymalin – Restores immune and endocrine balance for systemic skin regeneration.

38. GHK-Cu + Melanotan II (microdose) – Enhances skin tone, reduces photodamage, and boosts melanin for UV protection.

39. GHK-Cu + Humanin – Protects skin from mitochondrial oxidative stress.

40. GHK-Cu + ALA (Alpha Lipoic Acid) – Enhances collagen synthesis and reduces photoaging.

41. GHK-Cu + DSIP + Epitalon – Sleep, pineal, and peptide repair for overnight dermal regeneration.

42. GHK-Cu + Glutathione (IV or topical) – Brightens skin and detoxifies environmental skin damage.

43. GHK-Cu + PDRN (Salmon DNA Topical/Inj.) – Wound healing and anti-inflammatory synergy in aesthetic procedures.

44. GHK-Cu + IGF-1 LR3 + CJC-1295 – Tissue regeneration stack for collagen and dermal density.

45. GHK-Cu + HA Filler Support Stack – Post-injection peptide combination to improve filler longevity and skin quality.

46. GHK-Cu + Acetyl Hexapeptide-8 (topical) – Reduces facial fine lines and wrinkle depth with consistent use.

47. GHK-Cu + TB-500 + Hyaluronic Acid – Rehydrates dry or thinning skin with peptide repair support.

48. GHK-Cu + IGF-1 LR3 + Follistatin – Hair regeneration protocol targeting follicular density and skin repair.

49. GHK-Cu + NAD+ + MOTS-c – Age-reversal triad that repairs oxidative and hormonal skin damage.

50. GHK-Cu + Copper Oral + Topical – Dual copper system to support elastin and collagen formation and hair growth.

Senolytic & Longevity Clearance Stacks

1. **FOXO4-DRI + Dasatinib + Quercetin (D+Q)** – Powerful senolytic combination to selectively eliminate senescent cells.

2. **FOXO4-DRI + Fisetin** – Promotes clearance of senescent cells and enhances cognitive longevity.

3. **Epitalon + FOXO4-DRI** – Combines telomere support with senescent cell apoptosis for lifespan extension.

4. **FOXO4-DRI + NAD+ Precursors (NR/NMN)** – Supports DNA repair and energy metabolism after senescent cell removal.

5. **Fisetin + Quercetin + Piperine** – Natural senolytic cocktail that enhances systemic cellular clearance.

6. **Rapamycin (low-dose) + FOXO4-DRI** – mTOR inhibition combined with senescent cell apoptosis for aging control.

7. **FOXO4-DRI + Humanin** – Mitochondrial peptide support for stress resilience after senolytic treatment.

8. **FOXO4-DRI + MOTS-c** – Improves mitochondrial health and insulin sensitivity after senescent cell removal.

9. Dasatinib + Quercetin + MOTS-c – Combines clearance with mitochondrial renewal and metabolic optimization.

10. Epitalon + Dasatinib + Quercetin – Pineal and immune support alongside senescent cell clearance.

11. FOXO4-DRI + GHK-Cu – Promotes tissue regeneration following clearance of aged or dysfunctional cells.

12. FOXO4-DRI + BPC-157 – Accelerates tissue healing post-senolysis in joints, skin, and GI tract.

13. Rapamycin (weekly) + NAD+ IV – Deep autophagy induction followed by mitochondrial energy restoration.

14. FOXO4-DRI + TB-500 – Regenerates soft tissue after senescent cell clearance, especially post-injury.

15. Dasatinib + Fisetin + Apigenin – Synergistic senolytic and anti-inflammatory stack.

16. Rapamycin + Epitalon – Autophagy induction and pineal longevity optimization.

17. FOXO4-DRI + LL-37 – Combats residual infection or inflammation after immune-related senescence clearance.

18. Fisetin + GHK-Cu – Skin and connective tissue regeneration post-senescence removal.

19. FOXO4-DRI + 5-Amino-1MQ – Targets senescence and boosts NAD+ metabolism through NNMT inhibition.

20. FOXO4-DRI + Thymalin – Restores immune regulation post-senolysis.

21. Dasatinib + Humanin – Enhances mitochondrial cleanup after senescent immune cell clearance.

22. FOXO4-DRI + Epitalon + NAD+ – Telomere extension, senolysis, and energy optimization.

23. Fisetin + MOTS-c + Pterostilbene – Natural polyphenol-based clearance with mitochondrial enhancement.

24. Dasatinib + C60 (carbon 60) – Oxidative stress reduction with cellular senescence clearing synergy.

25. Rapamycin + Resveratrol + NAD+ – Combines autophagy, sirtuin activation, and mitochondrial renewal.

26. FOXO4-DRI + DSIP – Improves sleep-dependent senescent clearance and neural detox.

27. Dasatinib + FOXO4-DRI + BPC-157 – Systemic senolysis and gut-joint repair.

28. Fisetin + GHK-Cu + MOTS-c – Anti-aging skin and hair stack following senolytic cycles.

29. Rapamycin + Fisetin + Epitalon – mTOR modulation with long-term cellular age control.

30. FOXO4-DRI + IGF-1 LR3 (timed) – Regenerative response post-senolytic treatment in muscle and tissue.

31. FOXO4-DRI + Thymosin Alpha-1 – Immune system recalibration post-clearance.

32. FOXO4-DRI + Selank – Reduces neuroinflammation and restores mood post-senescence removal.

33. Dasatinib + LL-37 + NAD+ – Pathogen clearance and immune reset after senescent immune cell removal.

34. Rapamycin + MOTS-c + NR – Autophagy, mitochondrial support, and NAD+ replenishment.

35. Dasatinib + Quercetin + Epitalon – Cellular age reversal in tissues including skin and bone.

36. FOXO4-DRI + P21 Peptide (cyclical) – Targets senescent cells and enhances neural regeneration.

37. Dasatinib + NAD+ + Pterostilbene – Improves detox and longevity signaling post-senolytic therapy.

38. FOXO4-DRI + BDNF Mimetics – Promotes synaptic regeneration following brain aging clearance.

39. Rapamycin + ALA + Fisetin – Promotes detox, antioxidant recycling, and deep cell cleanup.

40. FOXO4-DRI + Melatonin (night) – Supports autophagy and immune tolerance when sleeping.

41. Rapamycin + 5-Amino-1MQ + Humanin – Metabolic and muscle-preserving longevity stack.

42. Dasatinib + Epitalon + Thymalin – Longevity peptide protocol with deep immune rebalancing post-clearance.

43. Fisetin + Carnosine + GHK-Cu – Muscle and skin rejuvenation in anti-aging recovery post-senolysis.

44. FOXO4-DRI + MOTS-c + GHK-Cu – Rejuvenates mitochondria and skin after senescent clearance.

45. FOXO4-DRI + DSIP + Humanin – Brain detox, neuroprotection, and deep sleep recovery.

46. Dasatinib + Thymalin + MOTS-c – Immune and metabolic clearance with immune restoration.

47. FOXO4-DRI + BPC-157 + KPV Peptide – Gut, joint, and inflammation recovery following senolysis.

48. Rapamycin + AOD-9604 + NR – Weight or fat cell senolysis and metabolic resetting.

49. FOXO4-DRI + NAD+ + Glutathione – Senescent cell clearance with redox and energy support.

50. Dasatinib + Rapamycin + FOXO4-DRI (cycling) – Aggressive, research-stage full-body senescent clearance protocol.

Neuro-regeneration & Brain Repair Stacks

1. **Dihexa + Semax** – Enhances synaptic growth, long-term memory formation, and learning speed.

2. **Dihexa + P21** – Promotes neural stem cell regeneration and reversal of cognitive decline.

3. **Cerebrolysin + Semax** – Neurotrophic and neuroprotective combination for post-stroke or brain injury recovery.

4. **Cerebrolysin + P21** – Powerful regeneration stack for neuronal repair in neurodegenerative conditions.

5. **Semax + Selank** – Balances cognition, anxiety, and neurotransmitter function post-injury or chronic stress.

6. **Dihexa + Humanin** – Supports synapse regeneration and protects mitochondria and neurons.

7. **MOTS-c + Dihexa** – Combines metabolic resilience and cognitive restoration.

8. **P21 + NAD+ (IV or oral)** – Boosts neuron repair and bioenergetics in aging or injured brains.

9. **Dihexa + NAD+ + Epitalon** – Synaptic and mitochondrial regeneration with pineal rhythm restoration.

10. Cerebrolysin + NAD+ – Enhances neurogenesis and cellular energy in cognitive aging.

11. Epitalon + DSIP + Semax – Combines deep sleep, pineal restoration, and brain plasticity.

12. BDNF Mimetics + Dihexa – Stimulates brain-derived neurotrophic factor for lasting neural improvements.

13. P21 + IGF-1 LR3 – Drives neuron regrowth and axon repair post-trauma or degeneration.

14. GHK-Cu + Semax – Reduces neuroinflammation and boosts cognitive clarity and mood.

15. Dihexa + IGF-1 DES – Localized brain repair after TBI or neurological surgery.

16. Cerebrolysin + BPC-157 – Enhances brain-gut axis recovery and neurovascular integrity.

17. Dihexa + DSIP – Supports overnight brain recovery and memory consolidation.

18. P21 + MOTS-c – Neuroimmune repair and oxidative resilience in high-stress conditions.

19. Selank + NAD+ Precursors – Stress-adapted cognitive repair and memory boosting.

20. Humanin + DSIP – Protects the brain from metabolic and oxidative insult during restorative sleep.

21. Dihexa + Epitalon – Synaptic repair with circadian and neuroendocrine support.

22. Semax + BPC-157 – Neurovascular and mucosal repair for brain fog and cognitive fatigue.

23. Cerebrolysin + Humanin – Supports neurogenesis and anti-apoptotic effects in Alzheimer's models.

24. P21 + Epitalon + NAD+ – Triad for anti-aging cognitive repair and neural maintenance.

25. MOTS-c + NAD+ + Semax – Enhances energy, cognition, and neuroplasticity post-stress.

26. Dihexa + CJC-1295 + Ipamorelin – GH axis support for brain repair and tissue regeneration.

27. DSIP + Cerebrolysin – Sleep and neurotrophic support after brain injury or burnout.

28. P21 + GHK-Cu – Tissue remodeling and neural repair synergy.

29. Semax + Lion's Mane Peptide (experimental) – Promotes NGF and supports neuroplasticity.

30. Selank + TB-500 – Addresses neuroinflammation and central nervous tissue healing.

31. NAD+ + MOTS-c + Humanin – Mitochondrial neuro-rescue stack for cognitive aging.

32. Dihexa + Fisetin – Synaptic regrowth with senolytic brain inflammation clearing.

33. BPC-157 + Semax – Repair of neurovascular and enteric-brain damage.

34. P21 + DSIP + NAD+ – Sleep-enhanced neurorepair with energy replenishment.

35. GHK-Cu + IGF-1 LR3 – Regenerates injured brain tissue and boosts cognition.

36. Humanin + BDNF Mimetics – Neuroprotection and plasticity after metabolic or viral brain stress.

37. Selank + Epitalon – Brain-pineal axis restoration in stress-related cognitive decline.

38. Semax + IGF-1 LR3 + NAD+ – Peak neuro-performance and aging defense stack.

39. Cerebrolysin + GHK-Cu + Dihexa – Recovery protocol for neuroinflammation and memory loss.

40. Dihexa + P21 + MOTS-c – Cognitive rejuvenation and neuroimmune balance.

41. DSIP + Semax + BPC-157 – Brain healing, sleep quality, and gut-brain interface optimization.

42. IGF-1 LR3 + P21 + NAD+ – Anti-aging regeneration and neural remodeling in cognitive fatigue.

43. Cerebrolysin + Epitalon – Long-term neuroprotective and anti-aging brain support.

44. GHK-Cu + NAD+ + Dihexa – Neuronal DNA repair and cognitive function boosting.

45. MOTS-c + Epitalon + DSIP – Metabolic, pineal, and brain recovery during sleep cycles.

46. Selank + Humanin + NAD+ – Mitochondrial neuro-calming and stress resilience.

47. P21 + LL-37 + NAD+ – Brain-immune repair after infection or autoimmunity-triggered cognitive decline.

48. Dihexa + IGF-1 DES + DSIP – Targeted brain region regeneration during sleep.

49. BDNF Mimetics + Dihexa + Epitalon – Synaptic enhancement with anti-aging rhythm stabilization.

50. Semax + P21 + MOTS-c + NAD+ – Comprehensive neuro-regeneration and cognitive longevity stack.

Chapter 14: HPA Axis Optimization

The hypothalamic-pituitary-adrenal (HPA) axis is the central neuroendocrine system that orchestrates the body's response to stress. It integrates signals from the brain, immune system, and peripheral organs to regulate cortisol production and maintain homeostasis. When the HPA axis is in optimal condition, it allows individuals to adapt to environmental challenges, modulate inflammation, and sustain energy balance. However, physiological stressors – namely, chronic stress, poor sleep, nutritional deficiencies, and metabolic disorders – can dysregulate this system. These stressors can cause conditions such as adrenal fatigue, depression, anxiety, metabolic syndrome, and impaired immune function. HPA axis optimization, therefore, refers to interventions—behavioral, nutritional, pharmacological, and lifestyle-based—that restore balance to this system and improve its resilience.

Physiology of the HPA Axis

The HPA axis begins in the hypothalamus, where stress triggers the release of corticotropin-releasing hormone (CRH). CRH, in turn, stimulates the anterior pituitary gland to secrete adrenocorticotropic hormone (ACTH), which acts on the adrenal cortex and prompts cortisol secretion. Cortisol mobilizes glucose, suppresses nonessential functions such as digestion, and regulates immune responses. Feedback loops ensure cortisol levels return to baseline once the stressor subsides.

Disruptions at any level of this axis—whether due to chronic stress, inflammation, or metabolic insults—can produce maladaptive cortisol rhythms, characterized by a disruption of the natural diurnal curve (high in the morning, low at night). This dysregulation may result in blunted or reversed cortisol secretion that can manifest as fatigue, poor sleep, and reduced stress tolerance.

Principles of HPA Axis Optimization

Optimizing the HPA axis involves interventions that restore **cortisol rhythm**, enhance **resilience to stressors**, and support **neuroendocrine-immune balance**. They can be grouped into:

1. **Lifestyle interventions** – sleep hygiene, exercise, circadian alignment.
2. **Nutritional strategies** – adequate micronutrients, adaptogens, anti-inflammatory diet.
3. **Behavioral approaches** – stress management, mindfulness, cognitive-behavioral therapy.
4. **Medical and supplemental approaches** – pharmacological modulation, targeted supplementation.

Lifestyle Interventions

Sleep Optimization

Sleep is fundamental to HPA axis health. Poor sleep quality or circadian disruption elevates evening cortisol and weakens the morning cortisol surge. Effective strategies for restorative sleep include:

- Consistent sleep schedules that align with natural light-dark cycles.

- Limiting blue light exposure before bed.
- Creating sleep environments with minimal noise and light.
- Practicing relaxation techniques such as progressive muscle relaxation.

Exercise

Regular physical activity provides a hormetic effect on the HPA axis. Moderate aerobic exercise improves cortisol regulation and resilience, whereas excessive training can exacerbate dysfunction. Recommended guidelines include:

- At least 150 minutes per week of moderate-intensity activity.
- Incorporation of yoga and tai chi, which combine movement with parasympathetic activation.
- Avoid overtraining, particularly if you are already experiencing fatigue.

Circadian Alignment

Light exposure profoundly influences HPA axis function. Morning sunlight enhances cortisol awakening response, while darkness promotes melatonin secretion. Strategies to optimize circadian light exposure include:

- Exposure to natural light within an hour of waking.
- Minimizing artificial light at night.
- Aligning meals and activity with daylight to reinforce circadian signals.

Nutritional Strategies

Macronutrient Balance

Blood sugar fluctuations act as a stressor on the HPA axis. Diets rich in refined carbohydrates can cause insulin spikes, which may result in compensatory cortisol release. A balanced diet with complex carbohydrates, lean proteins, and healthy fats stabilizes glucose and reduces cortisol load.

Micronutrients

- **Magnesium:** Regulates CRH and ACTH release. Magnesium deficiencies are associated with anxiety and HPA overactivation.
- **Vitamin C:** Concentrated in adrenal glands, and in high demand during stress.
- **B vitamins:** Essential cofactors in neurotransmitter and cortisol synthesis.
- **Omega-3 fatty acids:** Modulate inflammation and improve stress resilience.

Adaptogens

Herbal adaptogens such as ashwagandha, rhodiola, holy basil, and ginseng have been shown to normalize cortisol rhythms and enhance stress resilience. Clinical studies suggest ashwagandha reduces cortisol and improves sleep in stressed adults.

Anti-Inflammatory Diet

Chronic inflammation perpetuates HPA axis activation. Diets rich in antioxidants, polyphenols, fiber, and phytonutrients (Mediterranean-style diet) support systemic anti-inflammatory pathways and reduce HPA burden.

Behavioral Approaches

Mindfulness and Meditation

Mindfulness practices downregulate the sympathetic nervous system and improve parasympathetic tone. Studies show that regular meditation lowers basal cortisol and enhances emotional regulation.

Cognitive-Behavioral Therapy (CBT)

CBT addresses maladaptive thought patterns that contribute to stress perception. By reframing stressors, CBT reduces CRH and ACTH activation, leading to more balanced cortisol output.

Breathing and Relaxation Techniques

Slow diaphragmatic breathing stimulates the vagus nerve, which counteracts HPA overactivity. Progressive muscle relaxation and biofeedback also promote parasympathetic dominance.

Medical and Supplemental Approaches

Pharmacological Interventions

- **Cortisol-lowering agents** such as metyrapone are used in hypercortisolism.
- **Antidepressants** (SSRIs, SNRIs) indirectly modulate HPA dysregulation associated with depression.
- **Glucocorticoid replacement** is used in adrenal insufficiency.

These require careful monitoring by clinicians due to risks of overcorrection.

Supplements

- **Phosphatidylserine**: Shown to blunt excessive cortisol responses.
- **L-theanine**: Promotes alpha brain waves and reduces stress-induced cortisol spikes.
- **Probiotics**: Gut microbiota influence HPA signaling via the gut-brain axis; certain strains reduce stress reactivity.

Clinical Applications of HPA Optimization

Stress-Related Disorders

Patients with anxiety, depression, or PTSD often exhibit HPA dysregulation. Targeted optimization strategies can complement psychotherapy and pharmacotherapy.

Chronic Fatigue and Burnout

Blunted cortisol rhythms are common in occupational burnout. Interventions such as structured rest, adaptogens, and circadian realignment are often effective.

Metabolic Disorders

HPA dysfunction contributes to insulin resistance, abdominal obesity, and hypertension. Dietary and exercise-based optimization helps restore metabolic balance.

Autoimmune and Inflammatory Conditions

Cortisol's role in immune regulation links HPA dysfunction to autoimmunity. Interventions that reduce stress load and inflammation improve disease outcomes.

Monitoring and Assessment

HPA axis function can be evaluated using salivary cortisol profiles, serum ACTH, or dexamethasone suppression tests. These assessments help guide interventions and track progress. Salivary testing across the day is particularly useful in assessing diurnal rhythm.

Future Directions

Research into HPA optimization is expanding into personalized medicine. Genomic profiling may help predict individual vulnerability to stress-related dysfunction, while digital health technologies (wearables, apps) track sleep, activity, and stress biomarkers in real time. Integrative approaches combining neuroendocrinology, psychology, nutrition, and lifestyle interventions represent the future of HPA axis management.

Chapter 15: Cellular Regeneration

Cellular regeneration is the body's intrinsic ability to repair, renew, and replace cells to maintain tissue homeostasis and recover from injury. This process is not only essential for survival but also forms the biological foundation for longevity, healing, and disease resistance. Advances in peptide science have positioned bioactive peptides as powerful modulators of regenerative pathways, offering therapeutic potential in anti-aging, chronic disease management, and performance medicine.

The Biology of Cellular Regeneration

Stem Cells and Progenitor Cells

At the core of regeneration lies the stem cell, characterized by its ability to self-renew and differentiate. Adult stem cells reside in niches within bone marrow, skin, muscle, and other tissues, and they act as reservoirs for repair. Progenitor cells, while more specialized, also contribute to replenishing damaged tissues.

The Cell Cycle

Regeneration requires cells to progress through the cell cycle: growth (G1), DNA replication (S), preparation (G2), and mitosis (M). Tight regulation ensures fidelity of DNA replication and prevents oncogenic transformation. Growth factors and signaling cascades orchestrate this cycle, and peptides can act as modulators within these networks.

Apoptosis and Senescence

Cellular regeneration does not solely refer to cell creation but also controlled elimination. Apoptosis removes irreparably damaged cells, while senescence halts division in cells at risk of malignant transformation. However, accumulation of senescent cells can impair regeneration, which highlights the balance required between renewal and clearance.

Mechanisms of Tissue Regeneration

Wound Healing Paradigm

Tissue repair follows three overlapping phases:

1. **Inflammation:** Recruitment of immune cells and release of cytokines.
2. **Proliferation:** Fibroblasts, keratinocytes, and endothelial cells expand to rebuild tissue.
3. **Remodeling:** Collagen deposition, angiogenesis, and scar maturation restore structure and function.

Organ-Specific Regeneration

- **Liver:** Exceptional regenerative capacity, mediated by hepatocyte proliferation and hepatic progenitors.
- **Skeletal Muscle:** Satellite cells drive muscle fiber repair after injury.
- **Skin:** Basal keratinocytes and dermal fibroblasts restore the epidermis and dermis.
- **Nervous System:** Traditionally limited, though neurogenesis in the hippocampus and olfactory bulb highlights potential for repair.

Peptides as Regulators of Regeneration

Peptides are short chains of amino acids that act as signaling molecules, hormones, or fragments of larger proteins. Their ability to interact with receptors and influence cellular processes makes them uniquely suited to guide regeneration.

Growth Factor Mimetic Peptides

- **IGF-1 (Insulin-like Growth Factor-1):** Stimulates proliferation and survival pathways, especially in muscle and connective tissues.
- **GH secretagogues (e.g., Ipamorelin, CJC-1295):** Elevate growth hormone and indirectly boosts IGF-1 and enhances systemic regenerative potential.

Wound Healing Peptides

- **BPC-157 (Body Protection Compound-157):** Promotes angiogenesis, collagen formation, and fibroblast activity. Preclinical data suggest accelerated wound closure and tendon healing.
- **Thymosin Beta-4 (TB-500):** Enhances migration of keratinocytes and endothelial cells, which in turn facilitates repair in skin and muscle.

Neuroregenerative Peptides

- **Semax and Selank:** Synthetic analogs with neuroprotective and cognitive-enhancing effects. Evidence suggests roles in neurogenesis and synaptic plasticity.

Mitochondrial Peptides

- **Humanin, MOTS-c, SS-31:** Mitochondria-derived peptides that regulate oxidative stress, apoptosis, and metabolic signaling. They support cellular resilience and regeneration.

Molecular Pathways Influenced by Peptides

PI3K/Akt/mTOR Pathway

mTOR, a master regulator of growth and survival, integrates nutrient signals and growth factors to stimulate protein synthesis. Peptides modulating IGF-1 or GH pathways activate this cascade, which promotes anabolic repair.

AMPK and Metabolic Regulation

Peptides such as MOTS-c activate AMPK, a key energy sensor, which optimizes mitochondrial function and enhances cellular repair under stress conditions.

Angiogenesis Signaling

BPC-157 and TB-500 influence VEGF (vascular endothelial growth factor) pathways, which encourages capillary sprouting and blood supply to regenerating tissues.

Anti-inflammatory and Antioxidant Effects

By reducing NF-κB activation and oxidative stress, peptides protect against cellular damage. This in turn creates a more favorable environment for regeneration.

Clinical and Translational Applications

Orthopedic and Sports Medicine

Athletes and individuals who are recovering from musculoskeletal injuries increasingly turn to regenerative peptides. BPC-157 and TB-500 show promise in accelerating tendon, ligament, and muscle repair, which reduces downtime after injury.

Dermatology and Aesthetics

Peptides are integrated into topical formulations for skin rejuvenation. Palmitoyl pentapeptides stimulate collagen synthesis. It reduces wrinkles and improves skin elasticity. Wound-healing peptides accelerate recovery after dermatological procedures.

Neurology and Cognitive Health

Neuroregenerative peptides hold potential for treating stroke, traumatic brain injury, and neurodegenerative diseases. Enhancing neuroplasticity and protecting neurons may mitigate cognitive decline.

Anti-Aging and Longevity Medicine

Age-related decline in regenerative capacity is linked to stem cell exhaustion, mitochondrial dysfunction, and chronic inflammation. Peptides that target these pathways may restore youthful regenerative potential, which offers tools for longevity-focused protocols.

Challenges and Ethical Considerations

Safety and Regulation

While peptides are generally well tolerated, questions remain about long-term safety, dosing, and off-target effects. Regulatory frameworks vary, with some peptides classified as investigational or research-only compounds.

Accessibility and Quality

Peptide therapies are often compounded, which raises concerns about purity and consistency. Clinicians and consumers must navigate sourcing carefully to ensure safety.

Ethical Use

Performance enhancement in sports raises ethical concerns, particularly with growth-promoting peptides. Balancing medical utility with fair practice remains a challenge.

Future Directions in Cellular Regeneration and Peptides

Personalized Peptide Protocols

Advances in genomics and metabolomics may allow tailoring of peptide regimens to individual biological needs; a great way to maximize regenerative benefits.

Combination Therapies

Integrating peptides with stem cell therapies, exosomes, or gene editing could create synergistic regenerative interventions.

Digital Health Integration

Wearables and biomarkers that track stress, sleep, and recovery could inform dynamic peptide protocols to optimize regeneration in real time.

Expanding Research

Large-scale clinical trials are needed to validate efficacy, establish safety profiles, and move peptide therapies into mainstream medicine.

Chapter 16: Neurogenesis

Neurogenesis, the process of generating new neurons from neural stem or progenitor cells, represents one of the most fascinating frontiers in neuroscience and regenerative medicine. For decades, it was assumed that the adult human brain was fixed, incapable of producing new neurons after early development. However, research in the late 20th century overturned this dogma. Research demonstrates that neurogenesis persists into adulthood, particularly in the hippocampus—a region critical for memory, learning, and emotional regulation.

Understanding neurogenesis provides valuable insights into brain plasticity, cognitive resilience, and potential therapeutic strategies for neurodegenerative and psychiatric disorders. Within the context of peptide science, several bioactive peptides play essential roles in regulating neural stem cell proliferation, differentiation, and survival. These capabilities position them as promising tools for cognitive enhancement and neurological repair.

The Biology of Neurogenesis

Neural Stem Cells

Neurogenesis begins with neural stem cells (NSCs), which reside in specialized microenvironments, or niches, within the brain. These cells have the capacity to self-renew and give rise to neurons, astrocytes, and oligodendrocytes. Two major neurogenic niches in the adult brain are:

1. **Subgranular zone (SGZ)** of the hippocampal dentate gyrus.
2. **Subventricular zone (SVZ)** lining the lateral ventricles.

Stages of Neurogenesis

1. **Proliferation:** NSCs divide to generate neural progenitors.
2. **Differentiation:** Progenitors commit to neuronal lineage.
3. **Migration:** New neurons travel to their target regions (e.g., hippocampus, olfactory bulb).
4. **Integration:** Immature neurons extend axons and dendrites, which form synaptic connections.
5. **Survival:** Only a subset of neurons survives long-term, influenced by environmental stimuli and trophic factors.

Functional Relevance

New neurons in the hippocampus contribute to learning, memory consolidation, and pattern separation (the ability to distinguish similar experiences). Impaired neurogenesis is associated with cognitive decline, depression, and neurodegenerative conditions such as Alzheimer's disease.

Factors Influencing Neurogenesis

Positive Influences

- **Exercise:** Aerobic activity increases hippocampal neurogenesis, partly via elevated brain-derived neurotrophic factor (BDNF).
- **Enriched environment:** Cognitive stimulation, social interaction, and novel experiences promote neuronal survival and integration.
- **Nutrition:** Omega-3 fatty acids, polyphenols (e.g., resveratrol), and flavonoids enhance neurogenesis.
- **Sleep:** Adequate deep and REM sleep supports hippocampal neuroplasticity.

Negative Influences

- **Chronic stress:** Prolonged cortisol release suppresses neurogenesis.
- **Aging:** Stem cell exhaustion and reduced trophic support diminish neurogenic potential.
- **Inflammation:** Proinflammatory cytokines impair neural stem cell proliferation.
- **Neurotoxins:** Alcohol, drugs, and certain medications reduce neuronal survival.

Peptides and Neurogenesis

Peptides act as signaling molecules that influence neurogenesis through modulation of growth factors, neurotransmitters, and intracellular signaling cascades.

Neurotrophic Peptides

- **BDNF-mimetic peptides:** BDNF is a key regulator of neurogenesis. Peptide analogs or modulators of its receptor TrkB enhance neuronal differentiation and survival.
- **NGF-derived peptides:** Nerve growth factor fragments promote neurite outgrowth and cholinergic function.

Synthetic Peptides in Clinical Research

- **Semax:** A heptapeptide derived from ACTH fragments. It enhances BDNF expression, improves synaptic plasticity, and protects against ischemic injury.
- **Selank:** An anxiolytic peptide with neurotrophic properties. It is shown to modulate monoamine systems and support hippocampal neurogenesis.

Endogenous Neuropeptides

- **Vasoactive Intestinal Peptide (VIP):** Promotes neuronal differentiation and survival.
- **Neuropeptide Y (NPY):** Increases neural progenitor proliferation in the hippocampus.
- **Oxytocin and vasopressin:** Influence social behaviors and may indirectly support neurogenesis through stress modulation.

Mitochondrial and Metabolic Peptides

- **Humanin and MOTS-c:** Mitochondria-derived peptides that enhance cellular resilience and reduce oxidative stress, and both create favorable conditions for neuronal survival.

Molecular Pathways Modulated by Peptides

PI3K/Akt and mTOR

These pathways drive the survival and growth of neural progenitors. Peptides acting through IGF-1 and BDNF mimicry activate these cascades, which enhances neurogenesis.

MAPK/ERK Signaling

Crucial for neuronal differentiation and synaptic plasticity, often upregulated by neurotrophic peptides.

CREB (cAMP response element-binding protein)

Activation of CREB promotes transcription of BDNF and other neurogenic genes. Peptides that enhance CREB signaling indirectly support hippocampal neurogenesis.

Anti-inflammatory Mechanisms

Peptides such as thymosin beta-4 reduce inflammation, which in turn protects the neurogenic niche from cytokine-induced suppression.

Clinical Applications

Cognitive Enhancement

By promoting hippocampal neurogenesis, peptides like Semax and Selank are explored as nootropics to improve learning, memory, and executive function.

Mood Disorders

Depression is associated with reduced hippocampal neurogenesis. Antidepressant effects of some peptides may partly derive from enhanced neuronal proliferation and survival.

Neurodegenerative Diseases

Peptide therapies hold promise for conditions such as Alzheimer's and Parkinson's, where neurogenesis and synaptic integration are compromised. Enhancing neuronal replacement may slow cognitive decline.

Recovery from Brain Injury

Stroke and traumatic brain injury trigger limited endogenous neurogenesis. Peptides enhancing the survival and integration of new neurons could improve recovery outcomes.

Lifestyle and Peptide Synergy

Neurogenesis is best optimized by integrating peptide therapy with lifestyle interventions:

- **Exercise plus peptides:** Aerobic activity combined with BDNF-mimetic peptides may synergistically enhance hippocampal plasticity.
- **Nutritional synergy:** Diets rich in omega-3s and polyphenols support the trophic actions of peptides.
- **Stress reduction:** Meditation and adaptogenic peptides reduce cortisol, which acts as a key barrier to neurogenesis.

Challenges and Future Directions

Limitations in Measurement

Assessing neurogenesis in humans remains difficult. It mostly relies on indirect imaging or postmortem studies.

Safety and Regulation

Long-term safety of neurogenic peptides requires rigorous clinical validation. Uncontrolled neurogenesis could pose risks of aberrant connectivity or tumorigenesis.

Personalized Medicine

Future strategies may combine genetic profiling with peptide interventions to tailor neurogenic therapies to individual vulnerabilities, such as age-related decline or stress-related suppression.

Combination Therapies

Pairing peptides with stem cell therapies, exosomes, or gene editing could amplify neuroregenerative outcomes.

Chapter 17: Powerful Therapeutic Cycles

Peptides are versatile molecules that act as signaling agents, which regulate cellular communication, repair, and growth. While individual peptides can be effective on their own, the greatest therapeutic value often emerges from structured peptide cycles—timed regimens that optimize efficacy, minimize side effects, and allow the body's natural systems to reset. Just as in strength training or pharmacology, strategic cycling creates opportunities for synergy, adaptation, and sustained progress.

The Rationale for Peptide Cycling

Continuous administration of a peptide can cause receptor desensitization, diminished returns, and potential side effects. Cyclic use, on the other hand, provides:

- **Enhanced receptor sensitivity:** Periods of rest prevent downregulation and maintain peptide responsiveness.
- **Safety margins:** Off-cycles give organs, particularly the liver and kidneys, a chance to recover.
- **Synergistic sequencing:** Different peptides can be layered or alternated for complementary effects.
- **Adaptation windows:** Biological systems integrate changes better when pulses of intervention are followed by rest periods.

Peptide cycles typically last between **4 to 16 weeks.** The duration depends on the therapeutic goal and specific peptides used.

Categories of Therapeutic Cycles

1. Neuroprotective Cycles

Neurodegeneration, stress, and cognitive decline can all be addressed with peptide-based neuroprotective cycles. The goal is to enhance brain resilience, promote neurogenesis, and protect against oxidative stress.

- **Core Peptides:**
  - **Semax:** Enhances BDNF expression and supports memory.
  - **Selank:** Provides anxiolytic and neurotrophic support.
  - **DSIP (Delta Sleep-Inducing Peptide):** Improves sleep architecture, which is critical for neuroplasticity.
- **Cycle Example (8 weeks):**
  - Weeks 1–4: Semax daily; Selank every other day.
  - Weeks 5–8: Add DSIP at night 3–4 times per week.
  - Followed by a 4-week rest period to consolidate benefits.

Outcomes: Improved mood stability, sharper memory, enhanced learning capacity, and better sleep quality.

2. Metabolic and Fat-Loss Cycles

For patients who are targeting body recomposition, peptides that regulate insulin sensitivity, lipolysis, and mitochondrial efficiency can be combined.

- **Core Peptides:**
  - **AOD-9604:** Stimulates fat breakdown and inhibits lipogenesis.
  - **MOTS-c:** A mitochondrial peptide that activates AMPK, improving energy metabolism.
  - **GLP-1 analogs:** Enhance satiety and glucose regulation.
- **Cycle Example (12 weeks):**
  - Weeks 1–6: AOD-9604 daily in the morning; MOTS-c 2–3 times per week.
  - Weeks 7–12: Maintain MOTS-c, and add GLP-1 analog weekly.
  - After 12 weeks, pause for at least 4 weeks to assess progress and reduce receptor fatigue.

Outcomes: Reduced visceral fat, improved energy levels, enhanced insulin sensitivity, and better appetite control.

3. Muscle Growth and Performance Cycles

Athletes and individuals in rehabilitation benefit from peptides that increase protein synthesis, recovery, and muscular endurance.

- **Core Peptides:**
  - **CJC-1295 with Ipamorelin:** Potent GH secretagogues that elevate IGF-1 for anabolic repair.

    - **IGF-1 LR3:** Directly stimulates muscle protein synthesis and satellite cell activity.
    - **BPC-157:** Enhances tendon and ligament recovery to support performance.
- **Cycle Example (12–16 weeks):**
    - Daily administration of CJC-1295/Ipamorelin at night.
    - IGF-1 LR3 post-workout 3–4 times per week during the first 8 weeks.
    - BPC-157 on workout days or as needed for injury recovery.
    - Follow with an 8-week rest period to normalize GH/IGF-1 balance.

Outcomes: Increased lean muscle mass, reduced injury downtime, and improved workout recovery.

4. Immune Modulation Cycles

Immune-balancing peptides may be beneficial for individuals with autoimmune conditions, chronic infections, and systemic inflammation. The aim is to **restore equilibrium**—not overstimulate.

- **Core Peptides:**
    - **Thymosin Alpha-1 (TA1):** Enhances innate immunity and antiviral defense.
    - **Thymosin Beta-4 (TB-500):** Modulates inflammation and promotes healing.
    - **LL-37:** An antimicrobial peptide with activity against bacteria, fungi, and viruses.
- **Cycle Example (6–8 weeks):**
    - Weeks 1–4: TA1 twice weekly; TB-500 weekly.

    - Weeks 5–8: Introduce LL-37 twice weekly while tapering TA1.
    - Rest cycle for 4 weeks before repeating if clinically indicated.

Outcomes: Stronger immune resilience, reduced infection frequency, and balanced inflammatory response.

5. Anti-Aging and Longevity Cycles

Peptide cycles designed for longevity focus on mitochondrial support, DNA repair, and systemic regeneration.

- **Core Peptides:**
    - **Epitalon:** Telomerase activator linked to longevity research.
    - **Humanin and MOTS-c:** Mitochondrial peptides that counter oxidative stress.
    - **GHK-Cu:** A copper peptide that supports skin, collagen, and organ repair.
- **Cycle Example (12 weeks):**
    - Epitalon nightly for 20 consecutive days, then stop.
    - MOTS-c 2 times per week throughout.
    - GHK-Cu topical or injectable 3 times per week.
    - After completion, a 2–3-month rest period ensures balance.

Outcomes: Improved skin health, increased energy, better sleep, and potentially extended healthspan.

Designing Safe and Effective Cycles

Principles to Follow

1. **Individualization:** No two patients are the same. Cycles must be tailored to goals, health history, and response.
2. **Monitoring:** Track biomarkers (cortisol, IGF-1, insulin sensitivity) and subjective metrics (sleep, recovery, mood).
3. **Duration:** Most cycles should not exceed 12–16 weeks, and they should be followed by rest phases.
4. **Synergy, not overload:** More peptides do not equal better results. Choose combinations with complementary—not redundant—actions.
5. **Medical oversight:** While peptides are generally well tolerated, supervision reduces risks of adverse events.

Example: Comprehensive Regeneration Cycle

For an individual who is recovering from musculoskeletal injury while managing stress and cognitive fatigue, a **multi-target cycle** may include:

- **CJC-1295/Ipamorelin:** To increase systemic repair.
- **BPC-157:** For tendon and ligament healing.
- **Semax:** To improve focus and memory during recovery downtime.
- **TA1:** To strengthen immunity under physiological stress.

Structured as an **8-week program**, followed by rest, this type of cycle addresses the body holistically. The cycle helps with repairing tissue, protecting cognition, and supporting the immune system.

Future of Therapeutic Cycles

The future of peptide cycling lies in **precision medicine**. With advances in biomarker tracking, wearables, and AI-driven analytics, cycles will increasingly be:

- **Data-driven:** Adjusted in real time based on recovery scores, sleep quality, or hormone levels.
- **Personalized:** Genetic and epigenetic testing will reveal which peptides work best for each individual.
- **Integrative:** Cycles may combine peptides with stem cells, exosomes, or nutraceuticals for synergistic repair.

Bonus Questions and Answers

(1) A patient with a long-standing history of neurodegenerative disorder is being treated with peptides. What is the significant advantage of peptides for such patients?

(A) They act precisely on cellular targets.

(B) They have a high toxicity rate.

(C) They are less specific than the traditional treatment modalities.

(D) Peptides have a very low efficacy.

(2) All of the following statements regarding peptides are correct except:

(A) Peptides can be naturally occurring or synthetically engineered.

(B) They share a similar composition with carbohydrates.

(C) Peptides are short chains of amino acids connected by peptide bonds.

(D) They are highly versatile molecules.

(3) A nurse discusses the role of peptides in cosmetic products with a patient concerned about aging. Which benefit should the nurse mention that is attributed to peptides in skincare?

(A) Peptides can only hydrate the skin, not produce anti-aging effects.

(B) Peptides are mainly used for sun protection and do not affect wrinkles.

(C) Peptides have no proven benefits in cosmetic applications.

(D) Peptides stimulate collagen production, which improves skin elasticity and reduces wrinkles.

(4) What defines the primary structure of a peptide?

(A) Its overall three-dimensional shape.

(B) Covalent bonds formed between cysteine residues.

(C) The linear sequence of amino acids from the N-terminus to the C-terminus.

(D) Weak attractions between nonpolar side chains.

(5) Which of the following best describes the secondary structure of a peptide?

(A) The sequence of amino acids.

(B) Alpha helices and beta sheets.

(C) The weak attractions between nonpolar side chains.

(D) The covalent bonds between cysteine residues.

(6) All of the following bonds help stabilize the tertiary structure of a peptide except:

(A) Hydrogen Bonds.

(B) Disulfide Bridge.

(C) Van der Waals Forces.

(D) Hydrophilic interactions.

(7) Which classification includes peptides that contain between two and twenty amino acids?

(A) Dipeptides.

(B) Tripeptides.

(C) Oligopeptides.

(D) Polypeptides.

(8) Desmopressin is a synthetic analog of vasopressin used for which of the following purposes?

(A) Treating diabetes mellitus by increasing insulin secretion.

(B) Managing central diabetes insipidus by enhancing water reabsorption in the kidneys.

(C) Stimulating the release of growth hormone in individuals with growth deficiencies.

(D) Reducing inflammation by inhibiting prostaglandin synthesis.

(9) A patient with diabetes is prescribed insulin. How does insulin exert its effects on cellular metabolism?

(A) It directly inhibits digestive enzymes in the gut.

(B) It binds to insulin receptors and activates the intracellular signaling pathways.

(C) It forms pores in cell membranes to increase permeability.

(D) It modulates immune responses through cytokine release.

(10) In the emergency OPD, a nurse monitors a patient receiving angiotensin-converting enzyme (ACE) inhibitory peptides for hypertension. What is the primary mechanism by which these peptides lower blood pressure?

(A) They activate the renin-angiotensin system.

(B) They enhance vasoconstriction throughout the body.

(C) They increase the production of angiotensin II.

(D) They block ACE activity.

(11) A patient seeks help with obesity management, and a nurse recommends peptide therapy. All of the following mechanisms of action are utilized by peptides to promote fat loss except:

(A) Appetite Regulation.

(B) Lipolysis activation.

(C) Increased insulin sensitivity.

(D) Suppressed basal metabolic rate.

(12) Which peptide improves insulin sensitivity and prevents excessive fat storage?

(A) GLP-1 receptor agonists.

(B) Glucagon.

(C) Growth hormone secretagogues (GHS).

(D) Epinephrine.

(13) A nurse educates a patient on the role of peptides in weight loss. Which statement best reflects the function of peptides in appetite regulation?

(A) Peptides increase hunger signals to promote energy intake.

(B) Peptides influence the hypothalamus to decrease caloric intake.

(C) Peptides inhibit all hormonal functions related to appetite.

(D) Peptides do not exhibit an effect on appetite.

(14) During a patient education session, the nurse explains the importance of the injection technique for GLP-1 receptor agonists. Which of the following statements regarding the administration of GLP-1 receptor agonists is correct?

(A) Use the same injection site each time.

(B) Refrigerate the medication and dispose of needles properly.

(C) Preparation of the injection site is not required.

(D) Patients can administer GLP-1 receptor agonists on a flexible weekly or monthly schedule.

(15) A patient on GLP-1 receptor agonists inquires about the expected common side effects. All of the following are common side effects except:

(A) Nausea.

(B) Diarrhea.

(C) Pancreatitis.

(D) Abdominal pain.

(16) A nurse explains to a patient about the use of Ipamorelin. Which of the following statements should they emphasize regarding its mechanism of action?

(A) It mimics ghrelin's effects to stimulate growth hormone release.

(B) It inhibits growth hormone release.

(C) It directly increases blood glucose levels.

(D) It reduces appetite by acting on the hypothalamus.

(17) A nurse prepares to administer CJC-1295. What timing will optimize this injection's effects?

(A) The morning.

(B) At night.

(C) Immediately before exercise.

(D) Any time of day.

(18) Which of the following side effects is commonly anticipated in a patient receiving CJC-1295?

(A) Headache.

(B) Water retention.

(C) Injection site reactions.

(D) Joint pain.

(19) Which of the following peptides is approved for reducing abdominal fat in patients with HIV-associated lipodystrophy?

(A) CJC-1295.

(B) Ipamorelin.

(C) AOD-9604.

(D) Tesamorelin.

(20) A nurse teaches a patient how to administer Tesamorelin. What is the best injection site for Tesamorelin?

(A) The thigh muscle for better absorption.

(B) The same injection site to avoid discomfort.

(C) Subcutaneously into the abdomen; avoid the navel area.

(D) The shoulder area.

(21) A healthcare practitioner prescribes BPC-157 to a patient recovering from a muscle injury. What benefit does BPC-157 provide in the context of muscle repair?

(A) It suppresses blood flow to damaged tissues.

(B) It stimulates angiogenesis and improves blood supply to the damaged area.

(C) It increases the breakdown of muscle fibers.

(D) It has no impact on tissue healing.

(22) A nurse discusses how peptides such as IGF-1 and IGF-1 LR3 enhance athletic performance. How do peptides improve muscle recovery after physical activity?

(A) They enhance cell communication, which speeds the repair and rebuilding of muscle fibers.

(B) They slow down the body's natural recovery mechanisms.

(C) They promote excessive muscle breakdown.

(D) They do not affect muscle recovery.

(23) Which peptide is particularly helpful for patients recovering from overuse injuries, such as tendonitis or ligament strains?

(A) BPC-157.

(B) IGF-1 LR3.

(C) Ibutamoren.

(D) Ipamorelin.

(24) A patient in rehabilitation after surgery uses CJC-1295 and Ipamorelin. What is the main advantage of this combination therapy?

(A) It suppresses growth hormone release.

(B) It stimulates Growth hormone (GH) release and minimizes side effects from other hormones like cortisol.

(C) It only aids in fat loss, not muscle recovery.

(D) It has no impact on muscle growth.

(25) A nurse educates a patient about the benefits of BPC-157 for chronic joint pain. Which key point should the nurse emphasize?

(A) BPC-157 is ineffective for any type of injury.

(B) BPC-157 only works for muscle injuries, not joint pain.

(C) BPC-157 supports tissue repair and speeds recovery from overuse injuries.

(D) BPC-157 should be avoided in all athletes.

(26) What additional advantage does Ibutamoren provide beyond stimulating GH and IGF-1 release?

(A) It suppresses the pain cycle.

(B) It improves sleep quality, which is critical for recovery and well-being.

(C) It suppresses insulin secretion.

(D) It is effective for fat loss.

(27) A patient experiences significant muscle soreness after intense workouts. Which peptide might be beneficial for this patient due to its anti-inflammatory properties?

(A) IGF-1 LR3.

(B) CJC-1295.

(C) BPC-157.

(D) Ibutamoren.

(28) A nurse advises a patient about when to administer peptides in relation to exercise. What should they emphasize to achieve optimal results?

(A) Peptides should be taken only on rest days to avoid side effects.

(B) Peptides taken shortly before or after workouts can prolong the anabolic state and enhance recovery.

(C) Peptides can be taken at any time during the day.

(D) Peptides should only be taken after workouts to be effective.

(29) Which of the following statements regarding a consistent administration schedule of CJC-1295 and Ipamorelin is correct?

(A) Consistency is critical to maintaining elevated GH levels and achieving optimal muscle repair and growth.

(B) Consistency is not important; peptides can be taken sporadically.

(C) Peptides should be taken only during rest days for best results.

(D) It is best to take peptides only when feeling fatigued.

(30) IGF-1 (Insulin-like Growth Factor 1) is responsible for which of the following functions?

(A) Regulating calcium levels in the blood.

(B) Increasing water reabsorption in the kidneys.

(C) Stimulating cell growth and proliferation.

(D) Acting as a neurotransmitter in the central nervous system.

(31) A nurse educates a group of older adult patients about the potential benefits of peptides like Epitalon. What key mechanism should the nurse explain regarding how Epitalon may promote longevity?

(A) It directly increases muscle mass.

(B) It activates telomerase.

(C) It enhances appetite and weight gain.

(D) It reduces blood pressure significantly.

(32) Which of the following statements regarding the effects of Epitalon on circadian rhythms in aging populations is correct?

(A) It normalizes melatonin secretion.

(B) It disrupts melatonin production.

(C) It does not affect circadian rhythms.

(D) It increases melatonin production excessively.

(33) Which long-term benefits are most likely to be observed with Epitalon treatment in older adult patients?

(A) Increased risk of age-related diseases.

(B) Immediate weight loss.

(C) Reduced overall mortality and incidence of age-related diseases.

(D) Increased energy levels.

(34) What is one of the primary functions of Thymosin Beta-4 (TB4) in cellular processes?

(A) It inhibits cell migration.

(B) It promotes apoptosis.

(C) It regulates actin for cytoskeletal integrity.

(D) It stimulates hormone production.

(35) Which type of tissue does Thymosin Beta-4 (TB4) help repair following ischemic damage?

(A) Epithelial tissue.

(B) Cardiac tissue.

(C) Connective tissue.

(D) Adipose tissue.

(36) GHK-Cu can enhance which of the following processes related to skin health?

(A) Melanin production.

(B) Collagen synthesis.

(C) Sebum secretion.

(D) Keratin formation.

(37) What is a significant benefit of GHK-Cu in terms of skin condition?

(A) It reduces blood flow to the skin.

(B) It promotes collagen degradation.

(C) It enhances skin elasticity and reduces wrinkles.

(D) It increases skin sensitivity to environmental factors.

(38) What is not a possible mechanism of action attributed to BPC-157?

(A) Accelerated healing.

(B) Anti-inflammatory properties.

(C) Improved blood flow to injury sites.

(D) Induced apoptosis in damaged cells.

(39) Epitalon mainly helps delay the onset of which diseases?

(A) Diabetes and obesity.

(B) Cardiovascular diseases.

(C) Neurodegenerative diseases.

(D) Cancer and age-related diseases.

(40) Which of the following genes does GHK-Cu mainly downregulate?

(A) Genes linked to tissue repair.

(B) Genes linked to oxidative stress.

(C) Genes associated with immune function.

(D) Genes related to muscle growth.

(41) Which type of harmful stress to the brain is addressed by peptides?

(A) Nutritional stress.

(B) Oxidative stress.

(C) Thermal stress.

(D) Mechanical stress.

(42) Which of the following statements regarding the effect of glutathione (GSH) in the brain is correct?

(A) It promotes oxidative stress.

(B) It is a neurotransmitter.

(C) It neutralizes reactive oxygen species (ROS) and supports mitochondrial function.

(D) It damages cellular structures.

(43) What common feature is usually associated with neurodegenerative diseases like Alzheimer's disease (AD) and Parkinson's disease (PD)?

(A) Increased levels of glutathione (GSH).

(B) Elevated antioxidant defense mechanisms.

(C) Enhanced mitochondrial function.

(D) Depletion of glutathione (GSH).

(44) How do peptides like vasoactive intestinal peptide (VIP) and thymic peptides affect microglial activation within the brain?

(A) They reduce microglial activation.

(B) They enhance microglial activation.

(C) They do not affect microglial cells.

(D) They promote excessive inflammation.

(45) A nurse educates a family about the role of amyloid-β plaques in AD. What key point should the nurse emphasize regarding these plaques?

(A) Amyloid-β plaques enhance neuronal communication.

(B) Amyloid-β plaques are harmless and do not affect brain function.

(C) Amyloid-β plaque accumulation disrupts neuronal communication and contributes to neurodegeneration.

(D) Amyloid-β plaques only appear in healthy brains.

(46) In a clinical study, a patient is treated with VIP to address cognitive decline. How does VIP contribute to neuronal health in AD models?

(A) VIP increases amyloid-β aggregation, which worsens the condition.

(B) VIP inhibits the formation of amyloid plaques.

(C) VIP does not affect amyloid plaques.

(D) VIP directly repairs damaged neurons.

(47) Which of the following statements on the mechanism by which peptides enhance cognitive performance is correct?

(A) They directly enhance memory.

(B) They directly influence neurotransmitter systems and neuronal plasticity.

(C) They lower stress levels.

(D) They enhance sleep patterns.

(48) Which cognitive functions does the peptide Semax mainly enhance?

(A) Motor skills and reflexes.

(B) Emotional regulation.

(C) Visual perception.

(D) Attention, learning, and memory.

(49) Semax enhances the expression of which of the following proteins to support neuronal health?

(A) Glutamate.

(B) Acetylcholine.

(C) Brain-derived neurotrophic factor (BDNF).

(D) Serotonin.

(50) Cerebrolysin is commonly applied in which of the following clinical conditions?

(A) Weight loss.

(B) Stroke recovery.

(C) Diabetes management.

(D) Gastrointestinal disorders.

(51) Which type of immune cells do lactoferrin-derived peptides mainly interact with to enhance phagocytosis?

(A) Red blood cells.

(B) Platelets.

(C) Eosinophils.

(D) Neutrophils and macrophages.

(52) Lactoferrin-derived peptides inhibit the overproduction of which of the following pro-inflammatory cytokines?

(A) IL-2 and IL-4.

(B) TNF-α and IL-6.

(C) IL-10 and IL-12.

(D) IFN-γ and TGF-β.

(53) Lactoferrin-derived peptides enhance the overproduction of which of the following anti-inflammatory cytokines?

(A) IL-4.

(B) TNF-α.

(C) IL-10.

(D) TGF-β.

(54) A patient receiving antimicrobial peptides (AMPs) expresses confusion about how they enhance their immune system. Which explanation is the most accurate?

(A) AMPs solely eliminate bacteria without affecting cytokine levels.

(B) AMPs enhance macrophage activity and improve pathogen clearance while balancing cytokine levels.

(C) AMPs only increase inflammation to fight infections.

(D) AMPs directly replace the need for vaccines to prevent infections.

(55) A healthcare team reviews laboratory markers for a patient undergoing immunomodulatory therapy with AMPs. Which laboratory marker should the nurse monitor to gauge the inflammatory response?

(A) Hemoglobin levels.

(B) Blood glucose levels.

(C) Inflammatory markers.

(D) Serum electrolytes.

(56) Which parameters should nurses monitor in patients receiving peptide-based immunotherapies?

(A) Signs of altered immune responses.

(B) Only changes in appetite.

(C) The color of the medication.

(D) The patient’s weight.

(57) Due to cytokine modulation by peptides, nurses should watch for which potential complication?

(A) Chronic inflammation or immunosuppression.

(B) Decreased appetite.

(C) Interrupted wound healing.

(D) Decreased muscle growth.

(58) Where in the body are naturally occurring AMPs called defensins mainly found?

(A) The bloodstream only.

(B) Epithelial cells and neutrophils.

(C) Muscle tissues.

(D) Adipose tissues.

(59) How does LL-37 affect the immune response, which makes it unique from other cathelicidins?

(A) It enhances chemotaxis and cytokine production.

(B) It destroys bacterial membranes.

(C) It neutralizes viral infections.

(D) It inhibits the production of immune cells.

(60) A nurse educates a patient with multiple sclerosis about peptide-based therapies. Which statement best describes how these therapies work?

(A) They completely suppress the immune system to prevent attacks on myelin.

(B) They mimic myelin epitopes to modulate autoreactive T-cell responses.

(C) They increase the production of autoreactive T cells to enhance immune function.

(D) They only address disease symptoms without targeting the underlying causes.

(61) A patient with rheumatoid arthritis considers peptide-based treatment. What is the primary benefit of this approach compared to conventional immunosuppressants?

(A) It specifically targets inflammation without broadly suppressing the immune system.

(B) It eliminates the need for any medication.

(C) It increases joint damage to stimulate healing.

(D) It requires multiple injections for continued effectiveness.

(62) A healthcare team manages a patient with type 1 diabetes. They implement immunomodulatory peptides. What is the expected outcome of this treatment?

(A) Increased destruction of pancreatic beta cells.

(B) Enhanced overall immune response against all pathogens.

(C) Regulated T-cell activity to reduce the autoimmune attack on beta cells.

(D) Completely halt insulin production by the pancreas.

(63) A nurse notes that a patient undergoing peptide-based therapy for rheumatoid arthritis experiences reduced joint inflammation. Which mechanism of action is mainly responsible for this effect?

(A) Induction of systemic inflammation.

(B) Suppression of autoreactive T-cell activation.

(C) Complete eradication of all T cells.

(D) Increased production of pro-inflammatory cytokines.

(64) When considering the future of autoimmune disease management, what is a significant advantage of peptide-based therapies?

(A) They are less effective than traditional immunosuppressants.

(B) They require lifelong treatment without any monitoring.

(C) They are only effective in the early stages of the disease.

(D) They provide disease-specific interventions that minimize side effects.

(65) What is the chief significance of Major Histocompatibility Complex (MHC) presentation in immune responses?

(A) It allows T cells to recognize and respond to antigens.

(B) It prevents all immune responses.

(C) It mainly activates B cells.

(D) It degrades all peptides in the body.

(66) Which pathway translates extracellular signals into gene expression changes in immune cells?

(A) NF-κB pathway.

(B) MAPK pathway.

(C) JAK-STAT pathway.

(D) TLR pathway.

(67) What is a major challenge that peptides face in immunotherapy related to their stability?

(A) Peptides are too large to enter cells.

(B) Peptides are prone to enzymatic degradation.

(C) Peptides are always effective without modifications.

(D) Peptides induce an immune response that is too strong.

(68) What is a key advantage of synthetic biology in peptide-based immunotherapy?

(A) It enables the design of peptides with enhanced immunogenicity and specificity.

(B) It eliminates the need for dosing adjustments.

(C) It makes the peptide synthesis process very complex.

(D) It reduces the effectiveness of existing therapies.

(69) How do self-assembling peptide nanoparticles contribute to vaccine strategies?

(A) They decrease antigen stability.

(B) They mimic viral structures to enhance antigen presentation.

(C) They require complex administration techniques.

(D) They only target a single immune pathway.

(70) Why is it important for nurses to understand the mechanisms of action for peptide therapies?

(A) To manage patient responses and provide education during treatment.

(B) To eliminate the need for patient consent.

(C) To focus solely on administrative tasks.

(D) To administer therapies without monitoring.

(71) Which of the following statements regarding the characteristics of peptide hormones compared to larger proteins is correct?

(A) They have longer half-lives.

(B) They are less specific in their actions.

(C) They generally have shorter half-lives.

(D) They do not require receptors.

(72) Why is the pulsatile secretion of hypothalamic-releasing hormones important?

(A) It prevents the degradation of hormones.

(B) It ensures that target cells do not become desensitized to constant stimulation.

(C) It allows for continuous stimulation of the pituitary gland.

(D) It increases the overall hormone concentration in the bloodstream.

(73) Which statement regarding the role of Growth Hormone-Releasing Hormone (GHRH) in the human body is correct?

(A) It binds to receptors on pituitary somatotrophs to promote GH secretion.

(B) It inhibits the secretion of GH.

(C) It directly replaces deficient GH in the body.

(D) It acts mainly on the adrenal gland.

(74) Which of the following is a synthetic analog of GHRH that can promote the release of GH in individuals with deficiencies?

(A) GHRP-2.

(B) Sermorelin.

(C) Ghrelin.

(D) Insulin.

(75) What is the significant advantage of using GHRPs over recombinant GH?

(A) They require daily injections.

(B) They have a longer half-life than recombinant GH.

(C) They are less effective in promoting growth.

(D) They preserve the natural feedback mechanisms.

(76) Which side effect should nurses anticipate and monitor in patients receiving peptide therapies for GH deficiency?

(A) Insulin resistance.

(B) Decreased appetite.

(C) Urinary retention.

(D) Decreased energy levels.

(77) Which of the following statements regarding the significant advantage of using GLP-1 analogs over traditional insulin therapy is correct?

(A) They require daily injections.

(B) They make gastric emptying rapid.

(C) They enhance insulin release only when blood glucose levels are elevated.

(D) They enhance glucagon secretion.

(78) Which of the following should be monitored regularly in patients receiving peptide therapies?

(A) Only weight.

(B) Blood glucose levels, weight, and cardiovascular parameters.

(C) Only cardiovascular parameters.

(D) Only blood glucose levels.

(79) What potential benefit do GLP-1 analogs provide beyond glucose control?

(A) Low risk of pancreatitis.

(B) Low risk of dental carries.

(C) Low risk of prostatic cancer.

(D) Weight loss and cardiovascular protection.

(80) What is the primary function of thyrotropin-releasing hormone (TRH)?

(A) To inhibit the secretion of thyroid hormones.

(B) To stimulate the anterior pituitary gland to secrete thyroid-stimulating hormone (TSH).

(C) To stimulate the thyroid gland to secrete thyroid hormone.

(D) To stimulate the parathyroid gland to secrete parathyroid hormone.

(81) What is the primary purpose of the TRH stimulation test in clinical practice?

(A) To measure blood glucose levels.

(B) To diagnose diabetes mellitus.

(C) To assess kidney function.

(D) To evaluate the integrity of the hypothalamic–pituitary–thyroid axis.

(82) Which of the following parameters should nurses evaluate in patients following a TRH stimulation test?

(A) Blood glucose levels.

(B) Thyroid function.

(C) Liver enzyme levels.

(D) Serum electrolytes.

(83) What hormone is released by the anterior pituitary in response to CRH?

(A) Cortisol.

(B) TSH.

(C) Adrenocorticotropic hormone (ACTH).

(D) GH.

(84) Which proteins help maintain skin structure and elasticity?

(A) Hemoglobin and myoglobin.

(B) Collagen, elastin, and keratin.

(C) Insulin and glucagon.

(D) Enzymes and hormones.

(85) What are the four primary categories of peptides based on their mechanisms of action?

(A) Signal peptides, carrier peptides, neurotransmitter-inhibitory peptides, and enzyme-inhibitory peptides.

(B) Structural peptides, functional peptides, signaling peptides, and transport peptides.

(C) Antioxidant peptides, anti-inflammatory peptides, carrier peptides, and enzyme-inhibitory peptides.

(D) Growth peptides, repair peptides, hydration peptides, and protective peptides.

(86) What role do signal peptides play in the skin?

(A) They are cellular messengers that direct fibroblasts to produce components of the extracellular matrix.

(B) They inhibit collagen synthesis.

(C) They serve as antioxidants in the skin.

(D) They provide hydration directly to skin cells.

(87) Which peptide is known for mimicking the action of natural opioid peptides to relax facial muscles?

(A) Pentapeptide-18.

(B) Palmitoyl Tripeptide-5.

(C) Rice-derived peptides.

(D) Soy oligopeptides.

(88) Which of the following statements regarding the primary action of enzyme-inhibitory peptides in skincare is correct?

(A) They prevent the degradation of collagen, elastin, and hyaluronic acid.

(B) They stimulate muscle contractions.

(C) They enhance melanin production.

(D) They increase skin surface temperature.

(89) A fifty-year-old patient asks about effective anti-aging products. After discussing various options, the nurse recommends a cream containing Matrixyl 3000. What is the primary benefit of this peptide?

(A) It provides immediate lifting effects.

(B) It stimulates collagen production and improves skin hydration.

(C) It provides sun protection.

(D) It acts as an exfoliant to remove dead skin cells.

(90) A patient with sensitive skin is interested in using a serum containing Matrixyl 3000. Which complementary product should the nurse recommend to enhance its effectiveness?

(A) A heavy oil-based moisturizer.

(B) A retinol cream.

(C) A clay mask.

(D) A broad-spectrum sunscreen.

(91) A patient in their forties considers using a serum containing Syn-Ake to address fine lines. What key information should the nurse provide regarding the expected outcomes of using this peptide?

(A) It will provide permanent results after the first application.

(B) It will eliminate all wrinkles immediately.

(C) It is only effective for deep wrinkles.

(D) Its effects are temporary and require consistent use for visible results.

(92) A patient expresses concern about the nature of Syn-Ake and asks if it is comparable to Botox. How should the nurse explain the difference?

(A) Syn-Ake provides a temporary muscle-relaxing effect without injections, while Botox requires injections.

(B) Syn-Ake is a permanent injectable product, while Botox is a topical cream.

(C) Both Syn-Ake and Botox are permanent solutions to wrinkles.

(D) Syn-Ake is more effective than Botox in treating deep wrinkles.

(93) A patient is concerned about dark spots on their skin and is interested in using a product containing Tetrapeptide-30. What is the primary action of this peptide?

(A) It increases melanin production to even out skin tone.

(B) It inhibits tyrosinase activity and reduces melanin production.

(C) It acts as a physical exfoliant to remove dark spots.

(D) It provides immediate brightening effects.

(94) Which peptide is known to stimulate the release of gonadotropin-releasing hormone (GnRH)?

(A) PT-141.

(B) Kisspeptin.

(C) Oxytocin.

(D) Testosterone.

(95) What is the key difference between PT-141 and traditional treatments for sexual dysfunction like sildenafil (Viagra)?

(A) PT-141 targets the brain's sexual centers directly.

(B) PT-141 works through the vascular system.

(C) Sildenafil is more effective than PT-141.

(D) PT-141 is only for men.

(96) In which population has kisspeptin been shown to enhance sexual motivation and arousal?

(A) Only in men.

(B) Only in women.

(C) In both men and women.

(D) In older adult men.

(97) How does PT-141 (Bremelanotide) differ from traditional ED medications?

(A) It works solely on vascular mechanisms.

(B) It targets the nervous system instead of vascular pathways.

(C) It is only effective for women.

(D) It requires oral administration.

(98) What is the usual method of administration for PT-141?

(A) Oral tablets.

(B) Intravenous infusion.

(C) Subcutaneous injection.

(D) Topical cream.

(99) What is the first aspect that nurses should assess in patients with erectile dysfunction before they recommend PT-141?

(A) Their age and weight.

(B) The underlying causes of erectile dysfunction.

(C) Their previous sexual experiences.

(D) Their dietary habits.

(100) In which of the following clinical situations can PT-141 particularly benefit women?

(A) When there is a complete lack of sexual desire.

(B) During pregnancy.

(C) In cases of physical trauma.

(D) When arousal difficulties are due to psychological or hormonal factors.

(101) GHRP-6 is a growth hormone secretagogue that also stimulates the release of which neurotransmitter?

(A) Serotonin.

(B) Dopamine.

(C) Acetylcholine.

(D) GABA.

(102) CJC-1295 is a synthetic peptide known for its ability to:

(A) Inhibit cortisol production.

(B) Increase growth hormone secretion by extending the half-life of GHRH.

(C) Block dopamine receptors to regulate mood.

(D) Act as a direct agonist of insulin receptors.

(103) Ipamorelin is a selective growth hormone-releasing peptide known for its ability to:

(A) Inhibit cortisol production and suppress stress responses.

(B) Stimulate growth hormone release without significantly affecting cortisol or prolactin levels.

(C) Directly increase dopamine levels in the brain.

(D) Act as a competitive inhibitor of insulin receptors.

(104) Hexarelin is a synthetic growth hormone secretagogue known for its ability to:

(A) Act as a direct agonist of growth hormone receptors.

(B) Stimulate growth hormone release while also increasing prolactin and cortisol levels.

(C) Block the effects of ghrelin to regulate appetite and metabolism.

(D) Reduce the production of insulin-like growth factor 1 (IGF-1).

(105) Epitalon is a synthetic peptide known for its role in:

(A) Enhancing muscle growth and recovery through increased IGF-1 production.

(B) Stimulating growth hormone release by acting on the pituitary gland.

(C) Regulating telomerase activity to promote cellular longevity and anti-aging effects.

(D) Blocking cortisol receptors to reduce stress-related damage.

(106) BPC-157 is a synthetic peptide known for its ability to:

(A) Stimulate muscle hypertrophy by increasing testosterone production.

(B) Enhance healing and tissue repair by promoting angiogenesis and reducing inflammation.

(C) Block the effects of cortisol to prevent stress-related muscle breakdown.

(D) Act as a neurotransmitter to improve cognitive function and memory.

(107) TB-500 is a synthetic peptide known for its ability to:

(A) Promote wound healing, tissue regeneration, and cell migration.

(B) Increase testosterone levels for enhanced muscle growth.

(C) Act as a neurotransmitter to improve cognitive function and memory.

(D) Block the effects of cortisol to prevent stress-related muscle breakdown.

(108) PT-141 (Bremelanotide) is a synthetic peptide known for its ability to:

(A) Increase muscle mass by stimulating IGF-1 production.

(B) Enhance growth hormone secretion for improved athletic performance.

(C) Stimulate melanocortin receptors to improve libido.

(D) Reduce cortisol levels to prevent stress-related weight gain.

(109) AOD-9604 is a selective growth hormone-releasing peptide primarily known for its ability to:

(A) Increase muscle mass by directly stimulating IGF-1 production.

(B) Enhance cognitive function by acting as a neurotransmitter.

(C) Promote fat burning by stimulating lipolysis and inhibiting lipogenesis.

(D) Act as a vasodilator to improve blood flow and oxygen delivery.

(110) Tesamorelin is a synthetic peptide primarily used for:

(A) Stimulating insulin production to regulate blood sugar levels.

(B) Enhancing cognitive function and memory by acting on neurotransmitter receptors.

(C) Increasing growth hormone secretion to reduce visceral fat accumulation.

(D) Blocking cortisol release to prevent stress-induced weight gain.

Answers and Explanations

(1) (A) They act precisely on cellular targets.

Peptides are used to develop vaccines, such as in cancer immunotherapy and infectious disease prevention. Their ability to act precisely on cellular targets makes them a promising tool in the fight against complex diseases like neurodegenerative disorders and autoimmune conditions.

(2) (B) They share a similar composition with carbohydrates.

Peptides are short chains of amino acids connected by peptide bonds. They often consist of two to fifty amino acids. Although smaller than proteins, peptides share a similar composition and are essential building blocks in various biological processes.

(3) (D) Peptides stimulate collagen production, which improves skin elasticity and reduces wrinkles.

In cosmetics, peptides are incorporated into anti-aging products because they stimulate collagen production, improve skin elasticity, and reduce wrinkles.

(4) (C) The linear sequence of amino acids from the N-terminus to the C-terminus.

The primary structure is the linear sequence of amino acids in a peptide chain, described from the N-terminus (the end with a free amino group) to the C-terminus (the end with a free carboxyl group). This sequence determines the peptide's basic function and characteristics. It also dictates how the peptide will fold and interact with other molecules.

(5) (B) Alpha helices and beta sheets.

The secondary structure is the localized folding patterns within the peptide chain.

- Alpha Helices: A coiled structure stabilized by hydrogen bonds between every fourth amino acid.
- Beta Sheets: A flat, sheet-like structure formed by hydrogen bonds between segments of the peptide chain that may be far apart in the primary sequence.

Secondary structures are mainly influenced by the hydrogen bond between the backbone atoms in the polypeptide chain.

(6) (D) Hydrophilic interactions.

The tertiary structure refers to the overall three-dimensional shape of a single peptide or protein molecule.

The following are influencing factors.

- Hydrogen Bonds: Interactions between polar side chains that can stabilize folded structures.
- Disulfide Bridges: Covalent bonds formed between cysteine residues that can stabilize protein structure.
- Van der Waals Forces: Weak attractions between nonpolar side chains that contribute to stability.
- Hydrophobic Interactions: Nonpolar side chains tend to cluster away from water, which influences how the peptide folds.

(7) (C) Oligopeptides.

Peptides are classified based on their size, which is determined by the number of amino acids they contain. They include:

- **Dipeptides** are composed of two amino acids linked by a peptide bond.
- **Tripeptides** consist of three amino acids.
- **Oligopeptides** contain between two and twenty amino acids, often involved in signaling and regulatory functions.
- **Polypeptides** comprise twenty to fifty amino acids; they can fold into functional proteins depending on their sequence and interactions.

(8) (B) Managing central diabetes insipidus by enhancing water reabsorption in the kidneys.

Desmopressin is a synthetic analog of vasopressin (antidiuretic hormone, ADH) that acts on V2 receptors in the kidneys. By increasing water reabsorption in the collecting ducts, it helps reduce excessive urine output in conditions like central diabetes insipidus, which results from a deficiency of endogenous ADH. Desmopressin is also used for certain bleeding disorders, such as von Willebrand disease, due to its ability to stimulate factor VIII and von Willebrand factor release.

(9) (B) It binds to insulin receptors and activates the intracellular signaling pathways.

Many peptides, such as hormones or neurotransmitters, act as signaling molecules that bind to specific cell surface receptors (usually G-protein-coupled receptors or receptor tyrosine kinases). Upon binding, they activate intracellular signaling pathways that regulate various cellular processes, such as metabolism, growth, and immune response. For example, insulin is a peptide hormone that binds to the insulin receptor, which triggers pathways that facilitate glucose uptake and metabolism in cells.

(10) (D) They block ACE activity.

Peptides can regulate the activity of enzymes as inhibitors or activators. They may bind to the enzyme's active or allosteric site, which alters its functionality. For example, angiotensin-converting enzyme (ACE) inhibitory peptides block ACE activity, which reduces blood pressure by preventing the conversion of angiotensin I to angiotensin II, a vasoconstrictor.

(11) (D) Suppressed basal metabolic rate.

Peptides regulate fat metabolism by interacting with hormonal pathways and signaling systems. The key mechanisms include lipolysis activation, improved insulin sensitivity, boosted basal metabolic rate (BMR), and appetite regulation.

(12) (A) GLP-1 receptor agonists.

Some peptides modulate insulin activity, which prevents excessive fat storage. For example, GLP-1 receptor agonists improve insulin secretion and reduce insulin resistance, which helps maintain stable blood glucose levels.

(13) (B) Peptides influence the hypothalamus to decrease caloric intake.

Certain peptides influence the hypothalamus to regulate hunger and satiety, which reduces caloric intake and supports long-term fat loss. Understanding these mechanisms is essential to educate patients on how peptides assist in weight loss and metabolic health.

(14) (B) Refrigerate the medication and dispose of needles properly.

Proper injection techniques include site rotation and preparation to minimize infection risk. Patients must also adhere to storage requirements (refrigeration) and proper disposal protocols for used needles. Additionally, timing considerations are critical. Patients should administer semaglutide on a consistent weekly schedule and be educated on missed dose protocols and potential food interactions.

(15) (C) Pancreatitis.

Common side effects of GLP-1 receptor agonists include nausea, vomiting, diarrhea, and abdominal pain. Rare side effects include pancreatitis and gallbladder disorders. These medications must be started at a low dose and gradually increased to improve tolerance. Healthcare workers should encourage hydration and dietary adjustments to manage gastrointestinal symptoms.

(16) (A) It mimics ghrelin's effects to stimulate growth hormone release.

Ipamorelin is a selective GH secretagogue that mimics ghrelin's effects to release GH. Its short half-life makes it ideal for controlled dosing. Elevated GH levels enhance lipolysis, which promotes fat breakdown and preserves lean muscle mass. It also improves tissue repair and metabolic function.

(17) (B) At night.

Administering CJC-1295 at night may optimize GH release due to its natural pulsing pattern during sleep. Timing can also be adjusted based on individual schedules and responses. Dosing usually involves subcutaneous injections, with specific regimens depending on individual patient needs and treatment goals. Common dosing may range from 1 to 2 mg per week, divided into multiple doses.

(18) (C) Injection site reactions.

Common side effects of CJC-1295 are injection site reactions (e.g., redness, swelling). Rare side effects include headaches, water retention, or joint pain. Healthcare workers must ensure proper injection techniques to minimize local reactions. They should also monitor for excessive fluid retention or signs of carpal tunnel syndrome.

(19) (D) Tesamorelin.

Tesamorelin is a synthetic analog of GHRH designed to stimulate growth hormone secretion. It is highly specific for GHRH receptors as it minimizes off-target effects. It acts on the hypothalamus and pituitary gland to increase GH release. This results in enhanced lipolysis, which specifically targets visceral fat stores. It also improves insulin sensitivity. It is approved for reducing abdominal fat in patients with HIV-associated lipodystrophy.

(20) (C) Subcutaneously into the abdomen; avoid the navel area.

Tesamorelin should be injected subcutaneously into the abdomen, but the navel area should be avoided. The injection site must be rotated to prevent localized irritation or lipodystrophy. It should be administered at the same time each day, preferably at night, to mimic the natural circadian rhythm of GH secretion.

(21) (B) It stimulates angiogenesis and improves blood supply to the damaged area.

BPC-157 is a synthetic peptide derived from a protein found in gastric juice. It improves blood supply to damaged tissues, which supports tissue repair and stimulates angiogenesis (the growth of new blood vessels). This action promotes healing and recovery.

(22) (A) They enhance cell communication, which speeds the repair and rebuilding of muscle fibers.

These peptides improve cell communication, which speeds up the repair and rebuilding of muscle fibers after physical activity. They enhance the body's natural recovery mechanisms, which makes them valuable for muscle rehabilitation and growth.

(23) (A) BPC-157.

BPC-157 is a synthetic peptide that promotes joint, tendon, and muscle healing. It accelerates fibroblast activity and stimulates collagen production, a key protein needed for the strength and structure of connective tissues. This peptide is particularly helpful for patients recovering from overuse injuries, such as tendonitis and ligament strains, as well as exercise-induced damage.

(24) (B) It stimulates Growth hormone (GH) release and minimizes side effects from other hormones like cortisol.

These two peptides are often used together because of their complementary effects on GH production. CJC-1295 stimulates the release of GH from the pituitary gland, while Ipamorelin helps enhance this release without affecting other hormones like cortisol, which can cause unwanted stress-related effects. This combination improves muscle recovery, supports fat loss, boosts energy levels, and promotes lean muscle growth.

(25) (C) BPC-157 supports tissue repair and speeds recovery from overuse injuries.

BPC-157 can speed tissue repair, which makes it an attractive option for athletes or active individuals who need to recover quickly. Nurses may encounter patients using BPC-157 to manage chronic joint pain or aid in injury recovery.

(26) (B) It improves sleep quality, which is critical for recovery and well-being.

Unlike other peptides that are injected, Ibutamoren is taken orally. It stimulates the release of both GH and IGF-1, which play key roles in muscle growth, fat loss, and recovery. Ibutamoren is particularly appealing to patients who want the benefits of increased GH and IGF-1 without injections. In addition to supporting muscle growth and fat reduction, it also improves sleep quality.

(27) (C) BPC-157.

Intense exercise often causes inflammation in the muscles and joints, which can result in soreness and slow recovery. Specific peptides, such as BPC-157, have anti-inflammatory properties that help reduce exercise-induced inflammation. This allows individuals to recover faster and train more frequently, which builds strength and endurance over time.

(28) (B) Peptides taken shortly before or after workouts can prolong the anabolic state and enhance recovery.

Peptides must be administered at the appropriate time to maximize their effects. Research suggests peptides taken shortly before or after exercise sessions can prolong the body's anabolic (muscle-building) state.

(29) (A) Consistency is critical to maintaining elevated GH levels and achieving optimal muscle repair and growth.

CJC-1295 and Ipamorelin are GH-releasing peptides. They are particularly effective when administered before or after workouts. This schedule helps maintain elevated GH levels for an extended period, which promotes muscle repair and growth during recovery.

(30) (C) Stimulating cell growth and proliferation.

IGF-1, or insulin-like growth factor 1, is a peptide hormone structurally similar to insulin. It promotes cell growth, differentiation, proliferation, and survival. IGF-1 mediates many of the anabolic and growth-promoting effects of growth hormone (GH).

(31) (B) It activates telomerase.

Telomeres are repetitive nucleotide sequences located at the termini of chromosomes. They serve as protective caps that maintain genomic stability. Each time a cell divides, its telomeres shorten. When they become critically short, it causes cellular senescence or apoptosis. This progressive shortening is a hallmark of aging and contributes to the decline in tissue function over time. Epitalon is a synthetic tetrapeptide (Ala-Glu-Asp-Gly) derived from the pineal gland. It has garnered attention for its potential anti-aging properties. One of its primary mechanisms is telomerase activation. This enzyme adds telomeric repeats to the ends of chromosomes, which counteracts telomere shortening.

(32) (A) It normalizes melatonin secretion.

Melatonin is pivotal in regulating circadian rhythms, and disruptions in these rhythms are linked to various age-related disorders. Animal studies indicate that Epitalon can regulate melatonin secretion, which normalizes sleep-wake cycles. Epitalon treatment restored the daily rhythm of melatonin production in aging rats and aligned it more closely with patterns observed in younger animals.

(33) (C) Reduced overall mortality and incidence of age-related diseases.

Clinical studies in humans have had promising results. In older adult patients, Epitalon significantly increased telomere length in blood cells, which indicates its potential to rejuvenate aging cellular populations. Moreover, long-term studies have reported that Epitalon treatment is associated with reduced overall mortality and the incidence of age-related diseases.

(34) (C) It regulates actin for cytoskeletal integrity.

Thymosin beta-4 helps repair and remodel the cytoskeleton, which provides structural support and mobility to cells. Actin is a protein vital for cytoskeletal integrity. TB4 regulates actin, which promotes cellular processes like migration, division, and repair.

(35) (B) Cardiac tissue.

Research shows that TB4 can effectively repair cardiac tissue following ischemic damage and support the regeneration of nervous tissue. These remarkable abilities can be used to help treat heart-related injuries and neurodegenerative conditions, where tissue recovery is often limited.

(36) (B) Collagen synthesis.

GHK-Cu is a copper-binding tripeptide that helps enhance skin health and overall tissue resilience. It stimulates collagen synthesis, which accelerates wound healing and ensures faster injury closure and better-quality tissue regeneration.

(37) (C) It enhances skin elasticity and reduces wrinkles.

GHK-Cu supports the repair of skin damage caused by environmental factors and aging. It restores skin elasticity and reduces visible signs of aging, such as wrinkles and sagging. However, its regenerative properties extend beyond cosmetic benefits, as it promotes the functional health of skin cells.

(38) (D) Induced apoptosis in damaged cells.

BPC-157 stimulates the production of growth factors and promotes angiogenesis (the formation of new blood vessels). This action is critical for wound healing and tissue repair. It enhances the expression of GH receptors in various cells, which helps regenerate tendons, muscles, ligaments, and bones.

(39) (D) Cancer and age-related diseases.

Research on rodents has demonstrated that Epitalon can reactivate telomerase, which maintains chromosomal stability. This activation helps delay the onset of age-related diseases such as cancer while enhancing immune system function. Epitalon's ability to influence these essential biological processes underscores its potential to address molecular aging.

(40) (B) Genes linked to oxidative stress.

Research reveals that the peptide GHK-Cu significantly influences genetic activity. It upregulates genes associated with tissue repair and anti-inflammatory responses, which facilitates the body's ability to recover and maintain optimal function. Simultaneously, GHK-Cu downregulates genes linked to oxidative stress, a key contributor to aging and cellular damage. These findings suggest that GHK-Cu can help preserve cellular integrity and combat the adverse effects of aging.

(41) (B) Oxidative stress.

Peptides are short chains of amino acids that are essential signaling molecules. They regulate numerous biological processes, such as brain function. Research has focused on their role in neuroprotection, cognitive performance enhancement, and the management of neurodegenerative diseases. The brain is particularly susceptible to damage from oxidative stress, inflammation, and toxic aggregates. Peptides exhibit several mechanisms that protect neurons and maintain brain health.

(42) (C) It neutralizes reactive oxygen species (ROS) and supports mitochondrial function.

Glutathione (GSH) is a tripeptide that is a cornerstone of the brain's antioxidant defenses. GSH neutralizes ROS, which prevents cellular damage and supports mitochondrial function

(43) (D) Depletion of glutathione (GSH).

Research shows that GSH depletion is a common feature in neurodegenerative diseases such as AD and PD. The administration of GSH precursors like N-acetylcysteine (NAC) has shown promise in restoring redox balance.

(44) (A) They reduce microglial activation.

Although acute neuroinflammation is a protective mechanism aimed at combating injury or infection, chronic or dysregulated neuroinflammation can cause neuronal damage, neurodegeneration, and disruption of CNS homeostasis. Chronic neuroinflammation is a hallmark of conditions like AD and amyotrophic lateral sclerosis (ALS). VIP and thymic peptides suppress microglial activation, which reduces the release of pro-inflammatory cytokines. This modulation of the inflammatory response protects neuronal integrity and promotes a healthier brain environment.

(45) (C) Amyloid-β plaque accumulation disrupts neuronal communication and contributes to neurodegeneration.

Amyloid-β (Aβ) plaques are extracellular deposits of aggregated amyloid-β peptides in the brain. They are hallmark pathological features of AD and are implicated in neurodegeneration. The accumulation of these plaques disrupts neuronal communication, triggers neuroinflammation, and contributes to synaptic and neuronal loss.

(46) (B) VIP inhibits the formation of amyloid plaques.

In AD models, VIP has demonstrated the ability to inhibit the formation of amyloid plaques, which are toxic to neurons. VIP interacts with amyloid precursors and prevents their aggregation, which reduces neuronal death and preserves cognitive function.

(47) (B) They directly influence neurotransmitter systems and neuronal plasticity.

Cognitive enhancements improve mental functions such as memory, attention, executive function, creativity, and decision-making. They use pharmacological, behavioral, and technological interventions and are used in clinical and non-clinical settings. Cognitive enhancement through peptides involves mechanisms that boost memory, learning, and attention. These effects stem from their ability to influence neurotransmitter systems, neuronal plasticity, and overall brain health.

(48) (D) Attention, learning, and memory.

Semax is derived from an ACTH fragment, and it enhances cognitive functions such as attention, learning, and memory. It is clinically used in some countries for cognitive enhancement purposes.

(49) (C) Brain-derived neurotrophic factor (BDNF).

Semax increases the expression of BDNF, which is a critical protein for neuronal health. BDNF helps support the survival of existing neurons and encourages the growth of new neurons and synapses.

(50) (B) Stroke recovery.

Cerebrolysin is a peptide mixture derived from brain proteins that supports neurogenesis and neuronal survival. It has clinical applications in stroke recovery and has been shown to improve cognitive function in older adults.

(51) (D) Neutrophils and macrophages.

Lactoferrin-derived peptides modulate immune cell activity by binding to specific receptors on neutrophils, macrophages, and natural killer (NK) cells. These interactions increase phagocytosis, cytokine production, and overall immune system activation.

(52) (B) TNF-α and IL-6.

Peptides can regulate cytokine expression, which influences both inflammatory and anti-inflammatory responses. For example, lactoferrin-derived peptides play a dual role as they balance pro-inflammatory and anti-inflammatory cytokines, which maintain immune homeostasis. These peptides inhibit the overproduction of pro-inflammatory cytokines such as TNF-α and IL-6, which are commonly associated with excessive immune responses that cause chronic inflammation and autoimmune diseases.

(53) (C) IL-10.

Lactoferrin-derived peptides enhance the secretion of anti-inflammatory cytokines like IL-10, which helps suppress excessive immune responses and promote tissue repair. IL-10 downregulates antigen-presenting cell activity and limits the production of pro-inflammatory mediators. This action prevents tissue damage and autoimmunity.

(54) (B) AMPs enhance macrophage activity and improve pathogen clearance while balancing cytokine levels.

AMPs exhibit broad-spectrum antibacterial, antiviral, and antifungal properties, which defend against pathogens. These peptides disrupt microbial membranes, neutralize toxins, and modulate immune cell responses.

(55) (C) Inflammatory markers.

A nurse must work closely with the healthcare team to monitor laboratory markers regularly (e.g., inflammatory markers) and adjust care plans as needed. This ensures that the immunomodulatory therapy achieves its intended benefits with minimal adverse effects.

(56) (A) Signs of altered immune responses.

Nurses should closely monitor patients receiving peptide-based immunotherapies for signs of altered immune responses, such as excessive inflammation or inadequate immune activation. They should note changes in vital signs, fever, or local reactions at the injection site.

(57) (A) Chronic inflammation or immunosuppression.

Peptides modulate both pro-inflammatory and anti-inflammatory cytokines. Nurses must be vigilant for symptoms of cytokine imbalance, which could result in complications such as chronic inflammation or immunosuppression.

(58) (B) Epithelial cells and neutrophils.

Defensins are found in epithelial cells and neutrophils. They disrupt pathogen membranes and activate immune cells to protect against bacterial and viral infections. They also enhance cytokine production, which supports an effective immune response.

(59) (A) It enhances chemotaxis and cytokine production.

Cathelicidins (e.g., LL-37) are potent antimicrobial agents that destroy bacterial membranes, inhibit biofilm formation, and neutralize endotoxins. LL-37 is particularly significant due to its dual role. It enhances chemotaxis and cytokine production, which directly eliminates pathogens while modulating immune responses.

(60) (B) They mimic myelin epitopes to modulate autoreactive T-cell responses.

Peptide-based therapies aim to restore immune balance by targeting autoreactive T cells. For example, synthetic peptide analogs mimic self-antigens to induce immune tolerance, which reduces autoimmune attacks. These therapies selectively modulate T-cell responses, which suppress autoreactive lymphocytes while preserving overall immune function. In multiple sclerosis, peptides that mimic myelin epitopes help reduce autoreactive T-cell activity, which prevents demyelination and preserves nerve function. This limits nerve damage and functional decline.

(61) (A) It specifically targets inflammation without broadly suppressing the immune system.

Peptide-based treatments for rheumatoid arthritis suppress the inflammatory response. They modulate T-cell activation, which reduces joint inflammation and slows disease progression. These therapies target immune cells that drive the inflammation and may have more tailored and effective relief.

(62) (C) Regulate T-cell activity to reduce the autoimmune attack on beta cells.

In type 1 diabetes, immunomodulatory peptides help balance immune responses against pancreatic beta cells. By preventing destructive immune activity, they have the potential to reduce disease severity and delay the onset of insulin dependence. By selectively regulating these responses, peptide therapies provide a way to address autoimmune attacks without broadly suppressing the immune system.

(63) (B) Suppression of autoreactive T-cell activation.

In rheumatoid arthritis, peptide-based treatments dampen the inflammatory responses that cause joint damage. These peptides modulate T-cell activation, which is a critical driver of joint inflammation. As a result, they reduce the severity of joint inflammation, alleviate pain, and help slow cartilage and bone degradation. This provides a more focused treatment strategy than conventional immunosuppressants.

(64) (D) They provide disease-specific interventions that minimize side effects.

Peptide-based therapies are an innovative approach that provides disease-specific interventions that may improve outcomes and reduce side effects compared to traditional therapies.

(65) (A) It allows T cells to recognize and respond to antigens.

Peptides are central to antigen processing and presentation. When bound to MHC molecules on the surface of antigen-presenting cells, these peptides are recognized by T cells, which determines whether an immune response is activated or suppressed. This selective presentation ensures that the immune system targets pathogenic antigens and avoids self-antigens, which refines the specificity and balance of T-cell responses. Specific peptides can be engineered to enhance this process, which makes them promising immunotherapy candidates.

(66) (C) JAK-STAT pathway.

Many cytokines signal through the JAK-STAT pathway, which translates extracellular signals into gene expression changes that drive immune responses. Peptides that mimic cytokines or act as inhibitors can regulate this pathway and modulate the balance between pro-inflammatory and anti-inflammatory signals. This control maintains immune homeostasis and ensures a measured response during infection or inflammation.

(67) (B) Peptides are prone to enzymatic degradation.

Despite their potential, peptide-based immunotherapies face several challenges, such as stability, delivery, and immune tolerance. Peptides are prone to enzymatic degradation, which reduces their efficacy before they reach their intended targets.

(68) (A) It enables the design of peptides with enhanced immunogenicity and specificity.

Synthetic biology is revolutionizing peptide-based immunotherapy. It enables the design of synthetic peptides with enhanced immunogenicity and specificity. Engineered peptides with modified amino acid sequences exhibit improved resistance to proteolysis, which ensures longer circulation times and sustained therapeutic effects.

(69) (B) They mimic viral structures to enhance antigen presentation.

Self-assembling peptide nanoparticles improve antigen stability and immune response, which advances peptide-based vaccine strategies. These nanoparticles mimic viral structures, which enhance antigen presentation and promote robust immune activation.

(70) (A) To manage patient responses and provide education during treatment.

Peptide therapies are often administered via injection or infusion, and their dosing may be adjusted based on the desired immunomodulatory effect. Nurses must follow established protocols to ensure that the correct dose is administered via the appropriate route.

(71) (C) They generally have shorter half-lives.

Peptides can rapidly modulate cellular function, which makes them ideal for fine-tuning endocrine processes. Unlike larger proteins, they generally have shorter half-lives, which ensures that their actions are swift and transient. This rapid turnover is significant in systems where a quick adjustment is needed, such as during the regulation of blood glucose or stress responses.

(72) (B) It ensures that target cells do not become desensitized to constant stimulation.

Peptide hormones are synthesized and secreted in a pulsatile manner. For instance, the secretion of hypothalamic-releasing hormones is tightly regulated to stimulate or inhibit downstream hormone production in the pituitary gland. This pulsatility ensures that target cells do not become desensitized to constant stimulation.

(73) (A) It binds to receptors on pituitary somatotrophs to promote GH secretion.

GH plays a pivotal role in normal growth, metabolism, and tissue repair. GH deficiency, whether congenital or acquired, can result in growth disorders in children and metabolic disturbances in adults. Therapeutic approaches using peptide analogs have focused on two main strategies: to stimulate the release of endogenous GH and replace the deficient hormone itself. GHRH is a hypothalamic peptide that binds to receptors on pituitary somatotrophs to promote the secretion of GH.

(74) (B) Sermorelin.

Synthetic analogs of GHRH (e.g., sermorelin) have been developed to stimulate GH release in individuals with deficiencies. These peptides mimic the structure and function of natural GHRH, which causes increased pituitary secretion of GH. By enhancing the body's GH production, GHRH analogs can promote more physiological growth patterns and metabolic balance than direct hormone replacement.

(75) (D) They preserve the natural feedback mechanisms.

Clinical studies have shown that GHRPs can augment GH release and may also improve the pulsatility of GH secretion, which is critical for optimal metabolic effects. These peptides' therapeutic utility lies in their ability to restore a more normal endocrine milieu without daily injections of recombinant GH. Moreover, they preserve the natural feedback mechanisms that regulate hormone levels because they stimulate endogenous GH production.

(76) (A) Insulin resistance.

Nurses should regularly assess growth parameters, metabolic indicators, and signs of improved tissue repair in children and adults receiving peptide therapies. They should also monitor for side effects such as insulin resistance or edema.

(77) (C) They enhance insulin release only when blood glucose levels are elevated.

The gut secretes incretins in response to food intake. For example, GLP-1 binds to receptors on pancreatic β-cells, which causes an increase in intracellular cAMP. This activation promotes insulin secretion in a glucose-dependent manner. This means insulin release is only amplified when blood glucose levels are elevated. This mechanism enhances postprandial insulin secretion and reduces the risk of hypoglycemia.

(78) (B) Blood glucose levels, weight, and cardiovascular parameters.

Nurses should regularly monitor blood glucose levels, weight, and cardiovascular parameters to assess the effectiveness of peptide therapies in managing type 2 diabetes and metabolic syndrome. They should also watch for any adverse reactions, such as signs of hypoglycemia or gastrointestinal discomfort.

(79) (D) Weight loss and cardiovascular protection.

Modified analogs of GLP-1, such as exenatide and liraglutide, have been engineered to resist rapid enzymatic degradation. This prolongs their action and allows for less frequent dosing. These drugs have become a cornerstone in the management of type 2 diabetes. Their benefits extend beyond glucose control to include weight loss and cardiovascular protection.

(80) To stimulate the anterior pituitary gland to secrete thyroid-stimulating hormone (TSH).

TRH is synthesized in the hypothalamus. It stimulates the anterior pituitary gland to secrete TSH. TSH, in turn, acts on the thyroid gland, which prompts the production and release of the thyroid hormones T3 (triiodothyronine) and T4 (thyroxine). These hormones regulate metabolism, growth, and energy balance.

(81) (D) To evaluate the integrity of the hypothalamic–pituitary–thyroid axis.

In clinical practice, synthetic TRH has been administered during a TRH stimulation test to assess pituitary function. This diagnostic approach helps evaluate the integrity of the hypothalamic–pituitary–thyroid axis and identifies conditions such as secondary hypothyroidism or other pituitary dysfunctions.

(82) (B) Thyroid function.

Nurses should regularly assess TSH, T3, and T4 levels to monitor thyroid function, especially following TRH stimulation tests. Moreover, they should observe for clinical signs of thyroid dysfunction, such as changes in energy, weight, temperature sensitivity, or mood.

(83) (C) Adrenocorticotropic hormone (ACTH).

CRH is a hypothalamic peptide that helps control the body's response to stress via the hypothalamic–pituitary–adrenal (HPA) axis. Upon secretion, CRH binds to receptors on the anterior pituitary, which triggers the release of adrenocorticotropic hormone (ACTH). ACTH then stimulates the adrenal cortex to produce cortisol, which is a glucocorticoid that manages stress, modulates immune responses, and regulates metabolism.

(84) (B) Collagen, elastin, and keratin.

The demand for scientifically advanced skincare has led to the rise of peptides as one of the most effective cosmetic ingredients. Peptides are fundamental building blocks of proteins such as collagen, elastin, and keratin. These proteins help maintain skin structure, elasticity, and hydration. Unlike traditional skincare ingredients, peptides stimulate biological pathways involved in skin repair and rejuvenation.

(85) (A) Signal peptides, carrier peptides, neurotransmitter-inhibitory peptides, and enzyme-inhibitory peptides.

Peptides exert their effects through several biological mechanisms. They are categorized into four primary groups: signal peptides, carrier peptides, neurotransmitter-inhibitory peptides, and enzyme-inhibitory peptides. Each category has a unique function that contributes to skin repair, hydration, elasticity, and overall appearance.

(86) (A) They are cellular messengers that direct fibroblasts to produce components of the extracellular matrix.

Signal peptides act as cellular messengers that direct fibroblasts to produce essential components of the extracellular matrix (ECM), such as collagen, elastin, and glycosaminoglycans. These peptides mimic natural growth factors, which trigger regenerative processes that help maintain skin firmness and elasticity. Their function is particularly critical in anti-aging skincare, as they work to reduce the appearance of fine lines and wrinkles.

(87) (A) Pentapeptide-18.

Pentapeptide-18 mimics the action of natural opioid peptides. It provides a muscle-relaxing effect that maintains natural facial expressions. It helps smooth out dynamic wrinkles around the forehead and eyes without altering facial mobility significantly.

(88) (A) They prevent the degradation of collagen, elastin, and hyaluronic acid.

Enzyme-inhibitory peptides prevent the degradation of collagen, elastin, and hyaluronic acid, which protect the skin. These peptides block matrix metalloproteinases (MMPs), which are enzymes that break down structural proteins and contribute to skin aging. By inhibiting these enzymes, peptides help maintain skin integrity, hydration, and elasticity.

(89) (B) It stimulates collagen production and improves skin hydration.

Matrixyl 3000 is a well-researched anti-aging peptide that stimulates collagen production, improves skin hydration, and reduces the appearance of wrinkles. It mimics the skin's natural signaling mechanisms that enhance elasticity and firmness, which makes it a popular ingredient in anti-aging formulations.

(90) (D) A broad-spectrum sunscreen.

Nurses and skincare professionals should educate patients on the long-term anti-aging benefits of Matrixyl 3000. It is well-tolerated by most skin types, but individuals with sensitive skin should perform a patch test before use. Nurses should encourage patients to use complementary skincare products, such as broad-spectrum sunscreen, as they maximize the anti-aging benefits of Matrixyl 3000.

(91) (D) Its effects are temporary and require consistent use for visible results.

Nurses should inform patients that while Syn-Ake can help smooth expression lines, its effects are temporary and require consistent use for visible results. It also has potential contraindications for individuals with certain skin conditions or hypersensitivity to synthetic peptides.

(92) (A) Syn-Ake provides a temporary muscle-relaxing effect without injections, while Botox requires injections.

Syn-Ake is commonly incorporated into anti-aging serums and creams and targets fine lines and expression wrinkles. It is often used as a noninvasive alternative to Botox, as it provides a temporary muscle-relaxing effect without injections.

(93) (B) It inhibits tyrosinase activity and reduces melanin production.

Tetrapeptide-30 is a brightening peptide that inhibits tyrosinase activity, which is the enzyme responsible for melanin production. This effectively reduces hyperpigmentation, dark spots, and uneven skin tone.

(94) (B) Kisspeptin.

Kisspeptin is a neuropeptide that has emerged as a key regulator of sexual behavior, particularly in women. It stimulates the release of gonadotropin-releasing hormone (GnRH), which then triggers the release of reproductive hormones like luteinizing hormone (LH) and follicle-stimulating hormone (FSH).

(95) (A) PT-141 targets the brain's sexual centers directly.

Bremelanotide is another peptide that exerts its effects through the nervous system, although it operates differently from kisspeptin. PT-141 binds to melanocortin receptors in the brain, specifically MC1, MC3, MC4, and MC5. These receptors help regulate sexual desire and arousal. By stimulating melanocortin receptors, PT-141 activates neural pathways that increase sexual desire in both men and women. Unlike traditional treatments for sexual dysfunction, such as sildenafil (Viagra), which works through the vascular system, PT-141 directly targets the brain's sexual centers, which makes it an effective option for people with sexual arousal disorders.

(96) (C) In both men and women.

The stimulation of kisspeptin receptors in the hypothalamus increases sexual motivation, arousal, and orgasmic response in both men and women. This makes kisspeptin an exciting candidate for therapeutic interventions for those with hypoactive sexual desire disorder (HSDD) and other sexual dysfunctions.

(97) (B) It targets the nervous system instead of vascular pathways.

PT-141 activates melanocortin receptors in the brain, specifically MC1, MC3, MC4, and MC5 receptors, which are involved in sexual arousal and desire. This peptide bypasses the vascular pathways targeted by traditional ED medications and instead stimulates the central nervous system, which directly influences sexual desire and arousal.

(98) (C) Subcutaneous injection.

PT-141 is usually administered through subcutaneous injection, and it ensures patients are comfortable with this method of delivery.

(99) (B) The underlying causes of erectile dysfunction.

Nurses should assess the underlying causes of erectile dysfunction in patients before they recommend PT-141, as the peptide may not be effective for all causes of ED, particularly when vascular health is significantly compromised.

(100) (D) When arousal difficulties are due to psychological or hormonal factors.

PT-141 enhances sexual arousal in women by acting on melanocortin receptors in the brain. The peptide stimulates the central nervous system, which increases sexual desire and arousal in response to sexual stimuli. This mechanism is particularly beneficial for women who experience arousal difficulties due to psychological or hormonal factors.

(101) (B) Dopamine.

GHRP-6 (Growth Hormone Releasing Peptide-6) stimulates growth hormone release by acting on the pituitary gland. Additionally, it stimulates dopamine release, which plays a role in mood regulation, motivation, and appetite control.

(102) (B) Increase growth hormone secretion by extending the half-life of GHRH.

CJC-1295 is a growth hormone-releasing hormone (GHRH) analog that increases growth hormone (GH) secretion by extending the half-life of endogenous GHRH. It enhances GH release over a prolonged period, making it beneficial for muscle growth, fat loss, and recovery.

(103) (B) Stimulate growth hormone release without significantly affecting cortisol or prolactin levels.

Ipamorelin is a selective growth hormone secretagogue that stimulates GH release while minimally impacting cortisol and prolactin levels. This makes it a preferred choice for GH stimulation due to its reduced side effects and potential benefits in muscle growth, fat loss, recovery, focus, and mood enhancement.

(104) (B) Stimulate growth hormone release while also increasing prolactin and cortisol levels.

Hexarelin is a potent growth hormone-releasing peptide (GHRP) that stimulates GH secretion while also increasing prolactin and cortisol levels. It has a stronger GH-releasing effect than other GHRPs but may lead to higher prolactin and cortisol secretion, which should be considered when used for performance or therapeutic purposes.

(105) (C) Regulating telomerase activity to promote cellular longevity and anti-aging effects.

Epitalon is a synthetic tetrapeptide that stimulates telomerase activity, which helps maintain and extend telomeres—protective caps on the ends of chromosomes. By promoting cellular longevity, Epitalon is associated with anti-aging effects, improved sleep, and enhanced overall health.

(106) (B) Enhance healing and tissue repair by promoting angiogenesis and reducing inflammation.

BPC-157 (Body Protection Compound-157) is a synthetic peptide derived from gastric proteins that promotes healing, tissue regeneration, and anti-inflammatory effects. It enhances angiogenesis (formation of new blood vessels), making it beneficial for gut health, joint recovery, muscle repair, and injury healing.

(107) (A) Promote wound healing, tissue regeneration, and cell migration.

TB-500 is a synthetic version of thymosin beta-4, a peptide that plays a crucial role in cell migration, tissue regeneration, and wound healing. It promotes angiogenesis, reduces inflammation, and enhances recovery, making it popular for injury repair and muscle recovery.

(108) (C) Stimulate melanocortin receptors to improve libido.

PT-141 (Bremelanotide) is a melanocortin receptor agonist that influences the nervous system to enhance sexual arousal and libido. Unlike other sexual enhancement drugs that target blood flow (such as Viagra), PT-141 acts on the brain, making it effective for both men and women experiencing low sexual desire.

(109) (C) Promote fat burning by stimulating lipolysis and inhibiting lipogenesis.

AOD-9604 is a modified fragment of human growth hormone (HGH) that helps break down fat (lipolysis) and prevent the formation of new fat cells (lipogenesis). It is primarily used for weight loss and fat metabolism without significantly affecting blood sugar or growth hormone levels.

(110) (C) Increasing growth hormone secretion to reduce visceral fat accumulation.

Tesamorelin is a growth hormone-releasing hormone (GHRH) analog that stimulates natural growth hormone production, primarily used to reduce visceral fat, particularly in individuals with HIV-associated lipodystrophy. It helps improve body composition without significantly affecting blood sugar levels.

It is a hormone similar to the one normally released from the hypothalamus gland in the brain.

Access the audiobook, video tutorials and flash cards!

Scan the QR code below with your phone and you will be given a link to Google Drive where you can download the files.

If the QR code does not work for you, please contact mbenterprise2016@gmail.com and mention the title of this book.

Made in United States
Orlando, FL
10 November 2026

90498883R00223